Bridges Beyond *Sound*

Bridges Beyond Sound is an interactive videotape and companion workbook created to help students and teachers better understand Deaf culture and students with a hearing loss and build lasting friendships with classmates who have hearing impairments.

This instructional package has the following components:

Bridges Beyond Sound: An Instructional Video on Understanding and Including Students with a Hearing Loss
16-minute 1/2" VHS videocassette
Purchase of the videocassette includes one copy of the workbook.

Bridges Beyond Sound: An Instructional Workbook on Understanding and Including Students with a Hearing Loss
Additional copies of the instructional workbook can be purchased separately.

To order, contact Paul H. Brookes Publishing Co., Post Office Box 10624, Baltimore, Maryland 21285-0624 (1-800-638-3775).

Bridges Beyond *Sound*

An Instructional Workbook on *Understanding* and *Including* Students with a Hearing Loss

Corinne K. Jensema

with invited contributors
Debra Lennox and **Tina Downing-Wilson**

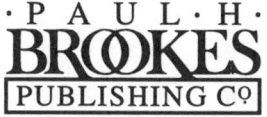

Baltimore • London • Toronto • Sydney

Paul H. Brookes Publishing Co.
Post Office Box 10624
Baltimore, Maryland 21285-0624

Copyright © 1996 by Corinne K. Jensema
All rights reserved.

Typeset by Signature Typesetting & Design, Baltimore, Maryland.
Manufactured in the United States of America by
BookCrafters, Chelsea, Michigan.

Initial funding for the preparation of this instructional package was provided by the U.S. Department of Education, Office of Special Education and Rehabilitative Services, under Grant #84.029K (PR/Award #H029K90078). Opinions expressed herein reflect the ideas and positions of the author and do not necessarily reflect the ideas or positions of the U.S. Department of Education; therefore, no official endorsement should be inferred.

ISBN 1-55766-226-6

Contents

About the Author ... vii
Foreword *Doin E. Hicks* ... ix
Preface ... xi
Introduction ... xiii
For the Reader ... xv
Acknowledgments ... xvii

Interactive Videotape Script and Instruction Guide
  Segment One ... 3
  Segment Two ... 15
  Segment Three ... 19

Applicable Teacher Supporting Materials
  T-1: Fact Sheet About Hearing Loss and
      People Who Have Hearing Impairments ... 25
  T-2: Questions Commonly Asked by Children
      About People Who Have Hearing Impairments ... 33
  T-3: Glossary of Terminology Related to Hearing Loss
      and People Who Have Hearing Impairments ... 36
  T-4: How to Use a TDD (TTY or TT) ... 43
  T-5: Interpreters for People with Hearing Impairments ... 47
  T-6: Selected Readings and Videotapes
      About Deafness and People Who Are Deaf ... 49
  T-7: State Organizations of and for the Deaf ... 52
  T-8: National and International Organizations of and for the Deaf ... 56
  T-9: Tips for Including Students Who Have
      Hearing Impairments in General Classrooms ... 66
  T-10: Tips for Evaluating Instructional Materials ... 68

Applicable Student Instructional Materials
  S-1: Pretest ... 71
  S-2: Facts and Myths About Deafness ... 77
  S-3: A World without Sound ... 81
  S-4: Fact Sheet About Hearing Loss and
      People Who Have Hearing Impairments ... 83
  S-5: Sample Audiogram ... 90
  S-6: Audiogram with Degrees of Hearing Loss ... 91
  S-7: Audiogram of Environmental and Speech Sounds ... 92
  S-8: How the Ear Works ... 93
  S-9: Diagram of the Ear ... 94
  S-10: Technology Used by People Who Have Hearing Impairments ... 96
  S-11: Connect-the-Dots ... 99
  S-12: Word Jumble ... 103

S-13: Communication Tips 106
S-14: Information Sheet on American Sign Language 107
S-15: American Manual Alphabet. 109
S-16: Fingerspelling. 110
S-17: Children's Books About People Who Are Deaf. 112
S-18: History of Deaf People in the United States. 114
S-19: Successful People with Hearing Impairments 119
S-20: Word Search: Successful People with Hearing Impairments 136
S-21: Children with and without
      Hearing Impairments Playing Together. 140
S-22: Crossword Puzzle 141
S-23: Posttest 147

Index 151

ABOUT THE AUTHOR

Corinne K. Jensema, Ph.D., has maintained a professional career in the field of deafness since 1971 as a teacher, school administrator, college professor, researcher, writer, consultant, journal editor, and impartial hearing officer. She has a bachelor of arts degree in English Education, a master of education in Deaf Education, a master of arts in Special Education Administration and Supervision from the National Leadership Training Program in Deaf-Blindness at California State University, and a doctor of philosophy in Special Education Administration and Supervision from Gallaudet University. Since 1986, Dr. Jensema has been President of the Institute for Disabilities Research and Training, Inc. (IDRT), a research, development, and consultation firm specializing in the field of disabilities.

Also contributing to this volume:

Debra Lennox, B.A., has served as Project Assistant on many of IDRT's research and program development projects involving individuals with hearing impairments. She graduated from the University of Maryland with a bachelor of arts degree in Hearing and Speech Sciences. Ms. Lennox has worked at the National Institute on Deafness and Other Communication Disorders as a management analyst and as a sign language interpreter. She has also worked in the public school system as a classroom interpreter.

Tina Downing-Wilson, B.A., served as Coordinator for the initial In-School Disability Awareness project funded by the U.S. Department of Education. She has served as a speech-language pathologist for children with autism and developmental disabilities, and as a staff trainer for paraprofessionals in human services. She managed five residential community living units for adults with developmental disabilities as an assistant director for the Washington County, Maryland, Association for Retarded Citizens. Ms. Downing-Wilson graduated magna cum laude with a bachelor of arts degree in Hearing and Speech Sciences from the University of Maryland and has 15 years of professional experience working with individuals with severe developmental disabilities.

FOREWORD

The "great melting pot" that once characterized America has taken on new meaning. No longer is it assumed that in order to "melt" into a uniquely American status one has to give up all current or former allegiance to other cultures or languages. We are gradually learning to appreciate the heritage that is uniquely American and at the same time cherish the diversity among us.

Interestingly, from the beginning, citizens with disabilities were never truly a part of the melting pot. Most were either kept at home or in institutions and schools for people with disabilities. Expectations of educators and families were often low and/or very narrow in scope. As the United States has become aware of civil and human rights issues and the value of cultures and diversity, so too have we become aware of the value of our citizens with disabilities. The fact is, if we live long enough, each of us will likely have a disability before we die.

A great deal has changed for citizens with disabilities since the mid-1960s. Large "special" institutions have given way to community-based models of support. "Special" schools have been downsized (some have closed) and changed in character, and most students with disabilities now attend public schools. The extent to which students with disabilities are fully included in classes with peers without disabilities varies considerably among school systems.

Among disabilities, deafness asks for an understanding that goes far beyond the recognition of loss of hearing. Often described as a "communication handicap," deafness is that and much more. Linguistic, cultural, and social implications often are particularly significant in understanding deafness. About 30% of people who are deaf have one or more educationally significant additional disabilities.

Unlike other disabilities, there is within the world of deafness at least one unique culture, known as Deaf culture. A large percentage of deaf people are members of this cultural and social group. Deaf culture flourishes in most countries of the world. There are smaller deaf groups who find support among deaf friends and colleagues who pride themselves in using oral methods (e.g., speech and speechreading) as their primary mode of communication.

Students who are deaf or hard of hearing have increasingly begun to enter the mainstream of public education. More than 80% are now attending public schools. Classroom settings vary widely—they range from self-contained to fully inclusive neighborhood settings. The trend toward full inclusion in the neighborhood setting is growing in popularity. In order for this to be successful for people who are deaf or hard of hearing, as well as for all people with disabilities, it is crucial that students, teachers, and other school personnel acquire a reasonable knowledge base about deafness and a sufficient level of skill in interacting with people who are deaf.

During the commencement program in May of 1995 at Gallaudet University, a deaf honor graduate gave a stirring and positive address to her fellow graduates, recounting her early perception of deafness. She spoke of her experience as a student in a public school and of the fact that until she was 14 years old she firmly believed that she would regain her hearing when she left school because she had never met an adult who was deaf and had never been given the opportunity to learn about the many accomplishments of deaf people.

The author of this volume and her colleagues have developed an instructional package, consisting of a workbook and videotape, that is outstanding. The job of teaching about hearing loss and deafness, from awareness and knowledge to having a positive attitude and skill and comfort in interaction, can be both satisfying and exciting. This package will enable a great number of teachers and classes to cross the bridge and stand on the firm footing of true understanding of deafness.

Doin E. Hicks
Professor Emeritus
Gallaudet University

PREFACE

The inspiration for this instructional package was derived from a recurring incident in our home—each year one of our children would come home from school and ask if he or she could bring Daddy to school for "show and tell." My husband, Carl, is not so unique in appearance or personality (although the latter may be arguable) as to warrant this kind of command performance, but he is profoundly deaf. The school curriculum in the county in which my family lives mandates that teachers address the issue of deafness with their students every few years; yet they are provided with few instructional materials (other than scientific information) with which to accomplish this task. My husband's presence reflects the teachers' need to put a human face and personal experience into the instructional process so that the children can understand that deafness is not summarized as an ear.

Although the impetus for this instructional package was Carl's annual show-and-tell reprise, keeping his schedule open was not a sufficient motivator to invest the kind of time that it took to develop this work. Among other professional occupations, I am an educational consultant for families and school systems that are encountering programmatic difficulties with students who have hearing impairments. With the passage of legislature and programs since the mid-1980s, more students with disabilities have been included in general education classes in the public schools, whether or not they are willing to be included. Even in the best circumstances—when the general classroom teacher, student, parents, and classmates are all deeply committed to "making it work"—there are frequently few tools to use as guidance to make implementation successful. Too often, the result is isolation for the student who has a hearing impairment, frustration for the teacher, and confusion for the student's peers. I witnessed a very poignant situation in 1994: For an entire high school day a deaf student was not once spoken to, nor did he speak to another person.

For inclusion to be successful for students who are deaf, critical steps must be taken. First, educators must recognize that students who are deaf are capable individuals and that these students consider themselves part of a culture. This culture is inextricably linked to the fact that they have a hearing loss. To ask many people who are deaf if they would rather be hearing is similar to asking an individual if he or she would rather belong to a different race, religion, or national origin. Intrinsic to including students with hearing impairments is the commitment to recognize them as a unique and valuable cultural group that should be represented, as are other cultural groups. Second, educators and classmates must have the skills to make inclusion work. It is not enough to have your heart in the right place. Inclusion cannot work through just smiles and pats on the back. All participants must have problem-solving skills to make sure that the student who is deaf is included in the communication loop.

This instructional package is designed to address these two goals. First, it provides teachers and students with information about the cultural history and practices of people who are deaf, it instills cultural pride in students who are deaf, and it assists teachers in choosing instructional materials that fairly and accurately present people who have hearing impairments. Second, it provides tips in nonverbal communication and practice in problem-solving situations in which communication or classroom procedures must be modified in order to fully include students who have hearing losses.

Recognizing the need of teachers to have an instructional package developed to teach students about people with hearing impairments, the U.S. Department of Education provided funding for the initial development of this instructional package under Grant #84.029K (PR/Award #H029K90078).

One of the benefits of having government funding for the development process was that we had the luxury of incorporating research about the product's utility. We were surprised to learn that not only did inclusion and general education students find it useful, but several students who are deaf who used it were inspired to do further research into their ethnic heritage. Several teachers reported that these students seemed less withdrawn in class and very actively participated in the implementation of this instructional unit. I sincerely hope that *Bridges Beyond Sound* can effect the same magic for your class.

～

We gave a copy of *Bridges Beyond Sound* to our neighborhood school. Carl is staying home a lot more.

INTRODUCTION

The purpose of this instructional package is to provide an educational model that presents positive images and attitudes toward children and adults who are deaf and hard of hearing in order to improve the quality of interaction between children with and without hearing impairments, particularly in general education settings. Teachers often have students with disabilities in their classrooms but are not provided with sufficient information to ensure that the students will be successfully integrated with their peers who do not have disabilities. School staff have begun to see the value of teaching units about ethnic groups so that children can be sensitized to the attributes, needs, and contributions of the groups. Teachers also need to have the instructional material resources available for teaching a unit on hearing losses.

Because students who are deaf and hard of hearing, like all students, rely on their families, schools, and peer groups for support, it is essential to raise school-age students' awareness, understanding, and, ultimately, comfort levels in interacting with children and adults who have hearing impairments to further enhance the social, moral, and academic development of all children and adults. In order for this to happen, educators need to do the following:

- Evaluate their own perspectives and instructional materials related to individuals who have hearing impairments.
- Become committed to actively acquiring information about disabilities that is both ethnographic and equitable.
- Be able to integrate this knowledge and belief system into their own teaching styles and curricula on a regular, ongoing basis.
- Have the capability to teach units about people with hearing losses, as teachers often do, to emphasize the attributes, rights, and contributions of a given race or culture.

The events that occurred during the spring of 1988 at Gallaudet University, the only institution of higher education in the world for people who are deaf, highlighted the fact that the needs and abilities of people who are deaf and hard of hearing in the United States continue to be unrecognized and unacknowledged. People with hearing losses routinely encounter situations in their social, professional, and educational lives that are patriarchal or charitable in nature. The fact that they require adaptive procedures to carry out common activities has caused many individuals to view them as deviant and, therefore, less than capable.

A situation involving Dr. I. King Jordan, the president of Gallaudet University, is a case in point. Dr. Jordan attended a state dinner during which there was a featured speaker. On the center of each table was a large floral centerpiece. Dr. Jordan placed his on the floor so that he could have a clear view of the sign language interpreter. His waiter placed the flowers back on the table. Dr. Jordan placed them on the floor a second time. The waiter again returned them to the table, stating that it is the established etiquette of service for all of the tables to be identically decorated. It took the intervention of the hotel manager for the flowers to be removed so that Dr. Jordan could have an unobstructed view of the interpreter. In this instance, Dr. Jordan's behavior was considered socially inappropriate to someone who had no understanding of the context of his actions.

It has long been acknowledged that developing positive attitudes is most successful when addressing children who have not yet had the opportunity to develop negative attitudes from older people. This instructional model will help teachers 1) develop their own knowledge, while increasing their students' knowledge and awareness of people with hearing impairments; 2) evaluate current educational curricula and materials for stereotyping and bias; and 3) acquire and use methods, media, resources, and materials for hands-on teaching of an ethnographic perspective of deafness.

FOR THE READER

Bridges Beyond Sound is an instructional package consisting of a workbook and an accompanying videotape. The workbook consists of three sections.

- Section I   Interactive Videotape Script and Instruction Guide
- Section II   Applicable Teacher Supporting Materials (all materials in Section II are labeled with a "T" for teacher supporting material)
- Section III Applicable Student Instructional Materials (all materials in Section III are labeled with an "S" for student handout)

Section I is divided into three segments, all of which utilize the script of the videotape. Segment One is intended to provide both you and your students with cultural, demographic, vocational, educational, sociological, and biological information about people who have a hearing loss. Segment Two presents typical situations in which there is a need to accommodate a student who is deaf; suggestions for accommodations in such situations are offered as well. In Segment Three, students are afforded opportunities to problem-solve situations for which accommodation is necessary. Time should be taken between each of the videotape segments to discuss the information presented, answer questions, problem-solve, and have your students use the handouts from Section III.

Sections I and II are designed to support and expand upon the information contained in the videotape. These sections include a range of information and are geared toward helping you provide instruction for children in grades 1 through 6. Interspersed throughout the script in Section I, at appropriate junctures, are questions to promote discussion with your students; suggested answers are also provided. Section II provides you, the teacher, with background information that will enhance your ability to lead this instructional unit.

The student handouts available in Section III were created to reinforce information learned from the videotape and related discussions. Each teacher should determine which of the materials are appropriate for each class and what should be included in the educational lesson plans. We recommend using the materials at the junctures specified in Section I or at the end of the associated videotape segments. All of the materials in Section III may be photocopied for educational purposes.

> We recommend that you view the entire videotape and read Sections I and II before utilizing this instructional package with your students. In this way, you will be thoroughly prepared to present this very important information to your students.

ACKNOWLEDGMENTS

The production of this instructional package would not have been possible without the tremendous assistance of three co-workers—Debra Lennox and Tina Downing-Wilson, who conducted background research and monitored and coordinated the details of this work, and Kathleen Schlor, who assisted in the fulfillment of editing requirements. They not only facilitated the development of *Bridges Beyond Sound*, but by their good natures, also rendered it an enjoyable task. Final production could not have been achieved without the able help of Theresa Donnelly and Mary Olofsson of Paul H. Brookes Publishing Co., who guided this work into publishable form. Finally, it must be noted that this work would not have been possible without funding from the Office of Special Education and Rehabilitative Services (OSERS) of the U.S. Department of Education that recognized the need to provide support to general education teachers who are facing the challenges of instructing deaf students in general education classrooms was substantial enough to warrant such an investment.

*To my husband, Carl Jensema, Ph.D., who is an early product of mainstreaming;
who, without the benefit of support services, reached the highest pinnacles of education;
and with whom I have created a bridge beyond sound.*

Bridges Beyond *Sound*

INTERACTIVE VIDEOTAPE
SCRIPT AND INSTRUCTION GUIDE

Segment One

The script of the Interactive Videotape is provided below. By reviewing it, you will have a better knowledge and understanding of the information and concepts contained therein. It will also cue you to appropriate times when the videotape should be stopped and discussions or other reinforcing activities initiated with your students.

> **APPLICABLE STUDENT INSTRUCTIONAL MATERIALS**
>
>  **Pretest**—The Pretest is included in the Student Instructional Materials and can be used to gauge your students' knowledge before instruction.

SCRIPT

Hello, I'm Gerald McRaney. You know just because a person has lost his or her hearing that doesn't mean they've lost the ability to be a good friend. If you're a hearing person, that's an important thing to keep in mind. And here's something else to know—there are 2 million people in the United States who have a hearing loss so severe that they're identified as being deaf. If you don't have a hearing problem, you might know someone who does—a parent, a grandparent, a brother, a sister, or a friend. Now, if you don't know someone with a hearing loss, I'd like to introduce you to someone very special who has something to say to you. Her name is Kathy Buckley.

Thanks, "Mac." Hi, I am Kathy, and I myself am hearing impaired. Now, in the video you're about to see we'll try to teach you a little about deafness and try to clear up some of the myths and stereotypes that hearing people have about deafness. Now, you might think there's some big problems that prevent communication between hearing and hearing impaired people. We're going to show you how to overcome those difficulties and give you a chance to see if you can solve those problems yourself.

Try to imagine a classroom without sound.

This is what the world of deaf people is like—in some ways, not much different from the world of hearing people, but in other ways nothing alike. Hearing people can never really know what it's like to live in that other world. But we're going to show you how to bridge the gap between the two worlds—to communicate, share thoughts and feelings, maybe even a joke or two. You'll see that, with a little work and understanding, you can learn to build bridges beyond sound.

Stop the tape

DISCUSSION

Questions to Ask Your Students

1. **Could you identify the individuals who have hearing impairments?**
   The scene you have just watched has been designed so that it is not easy to identify the individuals who have hearing impairments from those who do not.
2. **How could you tell who could hear and who could not?**
   Your students may have used different strategies for determining who has a hearing impairment and those who do not. Ideas cited may include wearing hearing aids, not being alerted to sound, and using sign language.

   The important point for you to emphasize to your students is that, for the most part, people who have hearing impairments do not look any different from people who can hear. They can be the same size, shape, color, age, and so forth. Especially from a distance, they will be indistinguishable from people who can hear. Deafness is a hidden disability. People who are deaf encounter a lot of misunderstanding because they are not immediately identified by strangers as people who have a disability.

APPLICABLE TEACHER SUPPORTING MATERIALS

| T-1 | Fact Sheet About Hearing Loss and People Who Have Hearing Impairments |
| T-2 | Questions Commonly Asked by Children About People Who Have Hearing Impairments |

APPLICABLE STUDENT INSTRUCTIONAL MATERIALS

S-2 **Facts and Myths About Deafness**
The second question may reveal familiar stereotypes and myths regarding hearing impairments. Some of the myths include that people who are deaf are less intelligent because of the way they speak or communicate, that people who are deaf are excellent speechreaders, that people who are deaf cannot get jobs or do not work, and so forth. You may want your students to do exercise S-2 at this point to gauge their knowledge and then redo it after the videotape is over to see how their answers have changed. Have your students evaluate how their own opinions have changed.

S-3 **A World without Sound**

SCRIPT

In the following scenes, see if you can identify who has a hearing impairment.

This time it's the boy carrying the ball.

Here's another chance to see if you can tell.

This time it's this man.

Now here's another chance—see if you can tell.

This one was tricky—in fact, this person is the only one without a hearing impairment.

NOTE

The family and friends in this last scene all have hearing impairments except for one female child. This is an example of *hereditary deafness*. These families pass on Deaf culture from parent to child. It may be interesting to note that the one child who does not have a hearing impairment has Down syndrome (a congenital syndrome that usually causes mental retardation). People who have hearing impairments can have children who have different, unrelated disabilities.

SCRIPT

That wasn't very easy, was it? That's because deaf people come in all sizes, ages, and colors. Many deaf people are older people, like some of your grandparents who lost their hearing when they got old. But others are children like you or adults like your parents. People can lose their hearing from diseases or accidents both before and after they are born. Some people who are exposed to loud noises at their workplaces can lose some of their hearing. Each person's hearing loss is different.

Stop the tape

DISCUSSION

Questions to Ask Your Students

1. **Does anyone in the class know someone who has a hearing impairment?**
   You may find that one or more of your students knows someone who has a hearing impairment. It is especially possible that it could be a grandparent. If a student does know a person who has a hearing impairment, ask him or her about that person.
2. **What kinds of noises do you think could cause you to lose your hearing?**
   There are many noises that can cause a temporary or permanent hearing loss. An important fact that everyone should be aware of is that whenever anyone experiences a temporary hearing loss or an intense ringing in his or her ears, it is a signal that the ear has been damaged. Most of the time this is only temporary, but repeated exposure to very loud noises will eventually result in a permanent loss. Types of noise that can damage a person's hearing include large machinery noises (e.g., bulldozers, factory machines, airplanes, helicopters, race cars, speedboats, trains), loud music (e.g., rock bands, using earphones and playing any music so loudly it hurts the ears), gunshots or military equipment (e.g., tanks, cannons, rifles, grenades, bombs), and firecrackers.

> **APPLICABLE STUDENT INSTRUCTIONAL MATERIALS**
>
>  **Fact Sheet About Hearing Loss and People Who Have Hearing Impairments**

SCRIPT

Some people have lost a little bit of their hearing. They may have trouble understanding people talk. These people are called *hard-of-hearing*.

People who have lost so much of their hearing that they can't hear people talk are called *deaf*.

There are several reasons that people with hearing losses speak differently. People who are hard-of-hearing usually can talk, but their voices may sound funny to you. When we learn language, we imitate the sounds we hear. Suppose someone is teaching you how to pronounce a new word.

If this was the way you heard things, could you understand what was being said? Could you repeat it?

MOTHER: Can you say "ball"?

> **Stop the tape**

DISCUSSION

Questions to Ask Your Students

1. **What word did the woman just say?**
   The mother said, "Ball." The audio is duplicating the way a person with a hearing loss might hear the word ball. A person with a moderate to profound hearing loss would only hear portions of the vowel sound "aw."
2. **Why do you think we all did not hear the same word?**
   Everyone in your class may not have heard the same word. This is because some people can hear only the vowel portion of the word and must depend on speechreading for the rest of the word. This is an important concept to be understood. It explains why people who have hearing impairments do not always understand what has been said, and it demonstrates for just a moment how a person with a moderate hearing loss experiences sound.

   At this point it might be helpful for you to discuss how your class can help a person who has a hearing loss receive the correct message. Ways of ensuring that the person with a hearing loss understands the message include writing down the message, pointing to the object you are talking about, repeating the most important words, and pantomiming the message.
3. **What sound would you miss if you had a high-frequency hearing loss? A low-frequency loss?**
   A high-frequency loss might cause you not to hear birds singing, air coming out of a balloon or tire, wind blowing, snakes hissing, some digital alerting sounds (e.g., microwave, watch), and certain consonants (e.g., *f, s, sh, ch, th*). A low-frequency loss might cause you not to hear fog horns, growling, motors, humming, and some vowels and consonants (e.g., *m, d, n, b, a*).
4. **How can you explain sounds to people who cannot hear them?**
   Use vibration, touch, and a mirror to show people who are deaf how certain speech sounds are made. (However, never put your hands on a person who is deaf or that person's hands on you without his or her permission, and do not put your hands in another person's mouth.) Vibration and touch also can be used to communicate environmental sounds, such as holding a balloon while music is playing because it is easier to feel the vibrations. Verbal descriptions work as well (e.g., the noise the freezer is making is like humming). Deaf people may have an idea what humming is because they can feel it in their own throats, or they can put their hands on your throat to feel the vibrations.

> **APPLICABLE TEACHER SUPPORTING MATERIALS**
>
> | | |
> |---|---|
> | T-1 | Fact Sheet About Hearing Loss and People Who Have Hearing Impairments |
> | T-2 | Questions Commonly Asked by Children About People Who Have Hearing Impairments |
> | T-3 | Glossary of Terminology Related to Hearing Loss and People Who Have Hearing Impairments |
>
> **APPLICABLE STUDENT INSTRUCTIONAL MATERIALS**
>
> | | |
> |---|---|
> | S-4 | Fact Sheet About Hearing Loss and People Who Have Hearing Impairments |
> | S-5 | Sample Audiogram |
> | S-6 | Audiogram with Degrees of Hearing Loss |
> | S-7 | Audiogram of Environmental and Speech Sounds |
> | S-8 | How the Ear Works |
> | S-9 | Diagram of the Ear |

SCRIPT

The sounds that people who are hard-of-hearing can hear are not clear. These sounds may be all they have to imitate.

People who are born deaf have trouble learning to talk because they have never heard speech at all, not even their own voices. Some deaf people don't speak at all.

You really can't always tell how much a person hears by the way they talk or if they sign.

One of these women can hear. Can you tell which?

If you guessed the woman on the left, you are correct.

Some people with hearing losses use hearing aids. Hearing aids make sounds louder for them, but the sounds they hear are not natural. They sound like machine-made sounds.

Stop the tape

DISCUSSION

Questions to Ask Your Students

1. **Do you know someone who wears a hearing aid?**
   If someone in the class tells you that he or she knows a person who uses a hearing aid, ask what that person is like and how he or she uses the hearing aid (e.g., for environmental sounds only, to hear speech). How does the hearing aid help that person, and what kind of hearing problems does the person still have even when he or she is wearing the hearing aid?

   Some of the responses may include statements such as, "The person uses the hearing aid for speech but still cannot hear like we can." Hearing aids squeal and make high-pitched noises when they do not fit tightly in the ear. This can cause distress or annoyance among the family and friends of a person who wears a hearing aid and for the person him- or herself who cannot figure out why everyone is nagging him or her about fixing the hearing aid.

2. **What do you think listening through a hearing aid sounds like?**
A hearing aid does not allow a person with a hearing impairment to hear like a person without a hearing impairment can. The sounds the person gets through the hearing aid are mechanical and cannot be perfectly calibrated to match the person's loss in each hearing frequency. This can make it very difficult for the person who has a hearing impairment to determine which sounds are important and which are not. For example, sounds like the hum of the refrigerator and clock radio may be transmitted at the same loudness as a speaker's voice, rather than at their natural decibel level.

3. **What do you think are the benefits and problems a person would have if he or she wore a hearing aid?**
A hearing aid may enable a person to pick up environmental sounds that he or she may not hear without the aid, which may be important for safety or informational reasons. In addition, a hearing aid may help others realize that a particular person has a hearing loss. As previously noted, hearing aids do not provide "true" sound. They need constant care—repairs, new ear molds (especially for children who grow and their ear size changes), and new batteries. They cannot be worn in the shower or while swimming and may cause discomfort when worn with eyeglasses and hats. Some people who have a hearing loss do not like the idea that hearing aids alert others to their deafness.

4. **Where could you go to get your hearing tested and to get a hearing aid?**
Hearing screenings for children are routinely done by schools and pediatricians. If problems with their hearing are detected, children may be referred to the department of audiology or ear, nose, and throat care in hospitals; clinics; speech and hearing or audiology private practices; and speech and hearing or audiology departments at universities. Hearing aids often can be ordered with a prescription through any of these centers or through a hearing aid dealer.

APPLICABLE TEACHER SUPPORTING MATERIALS

T-4   **How to Use a TDD (TTY or TT)**

APPLICABLE STUDENT INSTRUCTIONAL MATERIALS

S-10   **Technology Used by People Who Have Hearing Impairments**
S-11   **Connect-the-Dots**
S-12   **Word Jumble**

SCRIPT

If a person is deaf, a hearing aid may not be powerful enough to make sound clear enough for him or her to hear.

Some deaf people wear hearing aids just to help them know that sound is present and for safety reasons, like to let them know if a car is coming close to them.

Many people think that deaf people are good lipreaders or speechreaders—that is, they can tell what a person is saying just by watching the way the mouth moves. However, many words that sound different, look the same—"bye" and "pie," for example. Speechreading depends on training, practice, talent, and luck.

Stop the tape

DISCUSSION

Questions to Ask Your Students

1. **What is speechreading and why do some people with hearing impairments use this technique to communicate?**

    Speechreading is the skill of using vision alone to understand what is being said by another person. Speechreading is often called lipreading, but speechreading is a better term because more than just the lips are "read." In order to speechread, a person with a hearing impairment must learn to identify each sound by the shape of the speaker's mouth and other facial clues. Speechreading is very complicated. Many sounds in the English language are made using identical mouth movements (e.g., *m, p,* and *b* sounds) and cannot be distinguished visually. These sounds differ auditorially depending on whether they are voiced (e.g., *b*) or unvoiced (e.g., *p*), and where the voice is produced in the nasal cavity (e.g., *m*).

    Every person who has a hearing loss can speechread to some degree. The ability to speechread depends on a person's facility with the English language (if he or she is speechreading English), amount of residual hearing, training, talent, and luck. Children who are deaf typically speechread very little of what is said. It is estimated that the best speechreaders understand less than half of what is said to them.

    Additionally, a person's speechreading ability greatly depends on the speaker. For example, if a person with a hearing impairment has a high-frequency loss that prevents him or her from hearing high-pitched sound, he or she may be able to hear some sounds spoken by a man with a low voice but may not be able to hear any sounds from a woman with a high-pitched voice. Some speakers do not move their lips much when they speak; others have moustaches and/or beards that cover their lips; some people speak while they are eating; some have their hands or other obstacles over their mouths while they are talking; and some even turn away from the listener while they are speaking. These are all challenges that a speechreader must face every day. Take a look at all of the national television news anchors. Some of these people are considered to be the clearest articulators on television. However, if you turn off the sound on your set, you will find that it is very difficult to speechread what they are saying.

EXERCISE

Teach the class for 2 minutes without using your voice. Remember to use your lips as if you were speaking at a normal rate and without exaggerating your mouth movements. This will demonstrate to the class how complicated and difficult it can be to speechread. At the end of the 2 minutes, ask several children what they thought you said. Their responses will vary greatly.

APPLICABLE TEACHER SUPPORTING MATERIALS

| T-5 | **Interpreters for People with Hearing Impairments** |

APPLICABLE STUDENT INSTRUCTIONAL MATERIALS

S-4	**Fact Sheet About Hearing Loss and People Who Have Hearing Impairments**
S-13	**Communication Tips**
S-14	**Information Sheet on American Sign Language**
S-15	**American Manual Alphabet**
S-16	**Fingerspelling**

SCRIPT

Most deaf people find they are the only deaf person in their family. Usually deaf children have parents who can hear, and deaf parents have hearing children. [Dialogue.] Sometimes people have what we call *hereditary deafness*—this means it was handed down from parent or other relative to child in the same way that someone may inherit red hair or green eyes.

> **Stop the tape**

DISCUSSION

Questions to Ask Your Students

1. **Why was the father flashing the light?**
   The father was flashing the light to get the attention of his son who is deaf. This is a very common way to let a person who has a hearing loss know that you want his or her attention.

2. **Can you think of some other ways of getting a person's attention when he or she cannot hear?**
   - Tapping the person
   - Stomping on the floor
   - Waving your arms
   - Banging on a surface the person may be touching

3. **Does anyone in the class have a parent, grandparent, or sibling who has a hearing impairment?**
   If a student does have a relative who has a hearing impairment, ask the child what the person is like, how he or she gets that person's attention, and how that person communicates.

4. **How do families with members who have hearing impairments differ from families with no members who have hearing impairments?**
   Families that have a member who has a hearing impairment are atypical. The closest comparison may be a family with one member who is from a foreign country. Not only may that person not speak the language that the rest of the family speaks, but in a family with a member who is deaf, the "foreign" member cannot even learn the language the whole family speaks. These families must learn to use more than one communication system with the member who has a hearing impairment. They will have to use these dual systems their entire lives.

   Many people who have a hearing impairment never learn to communicate in English, and those who do learn English will always encounter barriers in the hearing world. The family must continually make an effort to include the member who has a hearing impairment in daily communications with people who can hear. They must learn alternative techniques to alert the person who has a hearing impairment and get his or her attention without chasing him or her all over the house. The homes of families who have a member with a hearing impairment often appear more noisy and chaotic than those of families that do not because of the extra physical activity that is involved in signing and physically contacting the member who has a hearing impairment.

   A deaf member of a hearing family may find it difficult to participate in some of the ethnic activities the other family members enjoy. For example, religious activities or occasions may not be signed, foreign languages may not be accessible, and music may be hard to appreciate. The member who is deaf may prefer to affiliate with Deaf culture, and the hearing members may feel uncomfortable joining in activities where no one is speaking.

5. **What are families like when all the members are deaf?**

Families in which all the members are deaf are in some ways like families in which all the members are hearing. If all members are hearing, there is typically no thought to accommodating a person who cannot hear. In families in which all the members are deaf, there is little thought to accommodating people who can hear. Such families' homes are usually designed to meet the needs of people who cannot hear—lights are used for alerting them to the telephone, the doorbell, alarm clocks, smoke detectors, a burglar system, or a baby crying. There is usually no stereo system or radio. The telephones all have telecommunication devices for the deaf (TDDs) by them, and televisions have closed-captioning features.

Families with all deaf members often prefer open floor plans because it allows everyone to have better visual access to each other. Noises that might irritate people normally are inconsequential. For example, it would not bother the children if the mother or father decided to vacuum or hammer a nail late at night. But, the family may be at risk of not heeding sounds that hearing families typically can hear, such as running water, the dog barking, a tea kettle boiling, the microwave beeping, the garbage disposal running, and so forth.

Parents who are deaf will pass along Deaf culture to their children. They tend to participate in Deaf culture events, such as sign language plays and social parties, picnics, and other gatherings. Everyday experiences are shared, and there is no need to compensate for one of the members because everyone is using the same communication system.

APPLICABLE TEACHER SUPPORTING MATERIALS

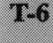 **Selected Readings and Videotapes About Deafness and People Who Are Deaf**

APPLICABLE STUDENT INSTRUCTIONAL MATERIALS

 Children's Books About People Who Are Deaf—Some of these books discuss life in a family that has a member with a hearing impairment and life as the only member with a hearing loss in a family.

SCRIPT

Usually, when deaf children have deaf parents, they feel they share a common culture, somewhat like Hispanic people, Jewish people, and Native Americans do. They share a special view of the world, traditions, history, and language.

Deaf people are very proud of their heritage. They are especially proud of other deaf people such as Linda Bove from *Sesame Street*, I. King Jordan, President of Gallaudet University, and Lou Ferrigno who plays the "Incredible Hulk," who have made important contributions to society and have become very well known. Deaf people have their own ways of expressing themselves in poetry, storytelling, and drama that have become very important to Deaf culture. Most of these use ASL and are transmitted from person to person or recorded on videotape since ASL is not a written language just like some American Indian languages.

Stop the tape

DISCUSSION

Questions to Ask Your Students

1. **What kind of traditions and history do you think people who are deaf share?**
   People who are deaf view the world in a special way, and this common experience helps them to develop a culture of their own. They share a language, sign language stories, and humor that can be uniquely appreciated because of their special way of experiencing life. They also share the history that chronicles the changes in attitudes of hearing people toward deaf people over the past few hundred years, the progress of deaf education, and contributions of people who are deaf.

2. **How do you think a person who is deaf views the world?**
   People who are deaf develop their view of the world based on their family, educational, peer, social, and occupational experiences, and on their experiences with interacting with the hearing world. They are a minority in society and share similar views that other minority groups share. Some people who are deaf believe that they are very limited by the way society views their disability. In other words, they believe that the disability itself is not as limiting as people's attitudes toward deafness and the consequent behaviors they manifest because of these attitudes.

APPLICABLE STUDENT INSTRUCTIONAL MATERIALS

S-18	History of Deaf People in the United States
S-19	Successful People with Hearing Impairments—12 short narratives about successful people with hearing impairments and pictures to color
S-20	Word Search: Successful People with Hearing Impairments

SCRIPT

Because most deaf children do not have deaf parents, many deaf children learn about Deaf culture from their other friends at school. People who consider themselves part of Deaf culture use a special language that is made with their hands and not spoken. This is called sign language. The sign language used in the United States is called American Sign Language or ASL.

Stop the tape

DISCUSSION

Questions to Ask Your Students

1. **Does anyone in the class know how to sign?**
   If a student in your class knows how to sign, ask the child to demonstrate his or her ability to the rest of the class. Many young children are very interested in signing and may have been exposed to sign language by watching *Sesame Street*, having a family member or friend who can sign, or receiving instruction in a prior class or service organization.

2. **Can anyone in the class understand the people in the videotape who are signing?**
   If any children in the class can understand American Sign Language (ASL), it is likely they are children of deaf adults (CODAs). There are some support groups around

the United States for CODAs because of their unique upbringing. For example, they may be asked to interpret for their parents at an early age and, although they are not deaf, may consider themselves part of Deaf culture.

3. **What is American Sign Language, and how is it different from the way we communicate?**

   ASL is a language that is made up of hand, face, and upper body movements that has its own grammar, vocabulary, syntax, and semantics. It is not English with signs tacked on, nor is it pantomime. It has no written form. Unlike a spoken language, it is not linear; that is, words are not made one at a time as they are in spoken language to render it auditorially efficient. They are made to be visually efficient. In a sign language, more than one concept may be presented simultaneously, similar to the way an eye takes in information.

   Consequently, when some people who are deaf attempt to write English, they may use incorrect language. A person may be fluent in ASL, but not English. He or she may be putting English in ASL order or confusing English words that look the same when speechread (e.g., shape/ship) or that share a sign (e.g., nice/clean).

4. **Is sign language universal?**

   No, sign language differs from place to place just as spoken language does. For example, the sign language used in Japan is not the same as the sign language used in the United States. The sign language used in the United States (ASL) has its roots in France, unlike the English language, which has its roots in England. Sign language differs from community to community in the same way that a person might have a Southern or New York accent and use slang, phraseology, and idioms unique to that geographic area. It is sometimes possible to tell which school for the deaf a person has attended by the signs he or she uses.

APPLICABLE STUDENT INSTRUCTIONAL MATERIALS

| S-14 | **Information Sheet on American Sign Language** |
| S-15 | **American Manual Alphabet** |

SCRIPT

You have seen ways that deaf people communicate with each other. "But," you may say, "I don't know sign language. How could I talk to a deaf person?" Before going on to the next part of the tape, see if you can make a list of all the different ways you can communicate with another person. If you really think about it, you will realize that people do not communicate *just* by talking.

Stop the tape

EXERCISE

Have your students make a list of different ways they could communicate with a person who has a hearing impairment. Have them pick an everyday kind of sentence like, "Where are your socks?" or "I am going to ride my bike," and express it in different ways. Some of the communication methods to try are the following:

- Mouthing the words
- Writing the sentence

- Drawing a picture
- Pantomiming
- Gesturing
- Signing
- Pointing

END OF SEGMENT ONE

Segment Two

SCRIPT

In the first segment we talked about deaf people, Deaf culture, and the special sign language that culturally deaf people use when speaking to each other. But, deaf people and hearing people need to communicate, too. Deaf people and hearing people share families, schools, workplaces, and public places. They may have important and also everyday things they want and need to say to each other.

At the end of the last segment, you were asked to make a list of different ways that people can communicate. Look at the list and think about which of these ways you could use with a deaf person and he or she could use with you.

CHILD: May I have a cookie, please?

You could say it with speech.

Or use sign language.

Or use a Signed English system.

You could write your message.

Or use pantomime to act it out.

Or point to things that you are talking about.

Deaf people can understand any kind of communication they can see or touch. Now, look at the list that you developed. Did you have some of the ways we just listed? Did you have any others?

Stop the tape

EXERCISE

Have your students compare the list that they wrote at the end of *Segment One* with the examples just given.

SCRIPT

In order to talk with deaf people, to get information across, we have to be creative at home, school, and on the playground. Look at these scenes and tell me what people did to find creative solutions to communicating.

BOY #1:   You want to play some basketball?

Deaf boy gestures that he cannot hear.

Hearing boy gestures, "Want to play?"

Stop the tape

DISCUSSION

Questions to Ask Your Students

1. **What did the boy do to communicate?**
   The boy pointed to the ball and tossed it a bit to indicate that he wanted to know if the other boy would like to join him in playing basketball. The type of ball and context (i.e., being on the playground by the basketball hoop) also were good indications of what the boy intended.
2. **What are some other things the boy could have done to communicate that he wanted the other boy to join him playing basketball?**
   Look for such suggestions as the following:

   - Point at the basketball hoop and at the other boy and himself.
   - Dribble and shoot the ball through the hoop and point at the other boy and then himself while using a questioning expression (e.g., raised eyebrows) or gesturing with shrugged shoulders and raised hands (i.e., implying "I don't know").
   - Write "Do you want to play?" on paper or in the dirt or sand.

SCRIPT

TEACHER: Good-bye—have a nice day.

What about this time? Can you pick out the creative solutions?

GIRL #1:   Hey, did you get the homework assignment?

GIRL #1:   Can you read my lips?

GIRL #2   (Shakes her head)

GIRL #1:   Did you get the homework assignment?...Homework assignment.

GIRL #2:   Yes. (nods) [Points to 1 through 9]

GIRL #1:   Okay.

Stop the tape

DISCUSSION

Questions to Ask Your Students

1. **What did the girl who could hear do to communicate?**
   The hearing girl tapped the girl who had the hearing impairment on the shoulder, faced the girl, asked the girl if she could read lips, pointed to her mouth, repeated what she said, and then pointed to the assignment on her paper.

2. **What else could the girl who could hear have done to communicate?**
   Look for such answers as the following:

   - Write down her question or point to her textbook and have a quizzical expression on her face.
   - Gesture with a shrug and arms upturned implying "I don't know."

3. **What should the girl have done differently?**
   She did not continue to face the girl who had a hearing impairment while she continued the conversation.

SCRIPT

As you can see, these people have found ways to work together even though one is deaf and one is hearing. With a little patience and ingenuity you can get through any difficulty and make a new friend.

You can learn many new things by making friends with people who are different from yourself. It can be very exciting and rewarding to meet people from other countries, different races, or other religions. Spending time with people who can't hear can open a whole new world. Not only can you learn more about Deaf culture and experiences, but you can also learn more about yourselves as hearing people.

END OF SEGMENT TWO

Segment Three

SCRIPT

In the last section, we talked about problem solving. You were asked to look at some scenes of people figuring out a creative solution to a problem. This time you'll have to figure out what to do yourselves. To give you an example, here's a situation.

Suppose you had a deaf student in your classroom who used an interpreter to follow along with what the teacher says. One day, the interpreter doesn't show up for the class. What can the students do to make sure the deaf student can follow the lesson?

Stop the tape

DISCUSSION

Questions to Ask Your Students

1. **What is an interpreter?**
   An interpreter is a person whose profession it is to change one language into another, so that two or more people who have different native languages can communicate. An interpreter is responsible for making sure that both parties understand each other. In other words, if a hearing person who uses English and a deaf person who uses ASL want to communicate, the interpreter must make sure that they both can understand each other. In a typical inclusive classroom, an interpreter helps the child who is deaf understand his or her classmates and teacher, while also helping his or her classmates and teacher understand him or her.
2. **TAKEN FROM THE VIDEOTAPE—What could we do to make sure a student who is deaf could follow the lesson if our interpreter were absent?**
   Look for the following answers:
   - One person could take notes for the student.
   - The student could sit next to the person taking notes so he or she could follow along.
   - The teacher could write important points on an overhead projector while talking.
   - The teacher and students could use more visual aids.
   - A peer could be assigned to sit with the student who is deaf and demonstrate what the teacher asked the class to do (e.g., "Open your books to p. 10").

> **APPLICABLE TEACHER SUPPORTING MATERIALS**
>
> **T-5** Interpreters for People with Hearing Impairments
>
> **APPLICABLE STUDENT INSTRUCTIONAL MATERIALS**
>
> **S-21** Children with and without Hearing Impairments Playing Together—A coloring page

SCRIPT

Now here's another one for you.

Suppose a deaf person asks you a question. Now, you could just shake your head and say, "I'm sorry, I don't know sign language." But, can you think of a better way to handle this?

Stop the tape

DISCUSSION

Questions to Ask Your Students

1. **TAKEN FROM THE VIDEOTAPE—What can you do if you did not understand something a deaf person said to you?**
   Some answers to look for include the following:
   - Knit your brows, look at the person, and shrug to indicate you do not understand.
   - Ask the person to repeat the sentence if his or her speech typically is clear.
   - Give the person a piece of paper and a pencil to write down what he or she is saying.
   - Ask the person to pantomime what he or she is trying to say.
   - See if anyone nearby can interpret for you.

SCRIPT

Suppose hearing and deaf people were ordering a pizza. You have to decide how big the pizza should be, what kind of toppings to order, thick crust or thin....How would you do it?

Stop the tape

DISCUSSION

Questions to Ask Your Students

1. **TAKEN FROM THE VIDEOTAPE—How could you decide as a group what everyone wants to order?**
   Look for such answers as the following:
   - Gesture with your fingers for the size and height of the crust.
   - Draw pictures of the toppings.

- Use your fingers to indicate how many pizzas or pieces of pizza.
- Draw a picture of a pizza divided into eight pieces and have each person write his or her initials on each piece to indicate how many pieces he or she wants to eat and what kind of pizza he or she wants.
- Point to choices on the menu.

SCRIPT

Suppose you can't hear and you are ordering food in a place where your number is called when your order is ready. How would you know when your order is ready?

Stop the tape

DISCUSSION

Questions to Ask Your Students

1. **TAKEN FROM THE VIDEOTAPE—How could a person who is deaf know that his or her order is ready?**
   Look for answers such as the following:
   - Look for an order to come up that is the same as what he or she ordered.
   - Tell the person taking the order ahead of time that he or she has to be physically contacted (e.g., tapped on the shoulder, visibly signaled).
   - Keep an eye on receipts or numbers if there is a system of sequential order-taking in which people have to take or are given numbers.

2. **How could you let the person with a hearing impairment know that his or her order is ready?**
   Look for answers such as the following:
   - Wave to him or her.
   - Tap him or her on the shoulder.
   - Bring the order to him or her.
   - Point to his or her number if a number system is used.

SCRIPT

During the course of this tape we learned a little about Deaf experience and culture. We also learned that when two people want to communicate, they both have to work at it and share the responsibility for getting their ideas across. We got a chance to be creative in finding ways to talk to people who can't hear and to understand what they want to say to us. [Dialogue.] These exercises have helped us to realize that when we are faced with a situation in which communication is difficult, we should take a little time and work it through, rather than run away from it. The efforts are so small and the rewards—oh, they're so great.

APPLICABLE TEACHER SUPPORTING MATERIALS

T-7	**State Organizations of and for the Deaf**
T-8	**National and International Organizations of and for the Deaf**
T-9	**Tips for Including Students Who Have Hearing Impairments in General Classrooms**
T-10	**Tips for Evaluating Instructional Materials**

APPLICABLE STUDENT INSTRUCTIONAL MATERIALS

S-22 **Crossword Puzzle**
S-23 **Posttest**

END OF SEGMENT THREE

Applicable Teacher Supporting Materials

T-1

FACT SHEET ABOUT HEARING LOSS AND PEOPLE WHO HAVE HEARING IMPAIRMENTS

DEFINITION

Deafness is defined by the Committee on Nomenclature, Conference of Executives of American Schools for the Deaf, as "that condition in which the sense of hearing is nonfunctional for the ordinary purposes of life" (1938, p. 1). The regulations for PL 101-476, the Individuals with Disabilities Education Act (IDEA) of 1990 states,

> 'deaf' means a hearing impairment which is so severe that the child is impaired in processing linguistic information through hearing, with or without amplification, and which adversely affects educational performance... [and] 'hearing impairment' means an impairment in hearing, whether permanent or fluctuating, that adversely affects a child's educational performance, but which is not included under the definition of 'deafness.' (*Federal Register,* 1992, p. 44801)

Defining a hearing loss is very difficult because so many variables are involved. This fact makes each person who has a hearing impairment unique. Age of onset, degree of hearing loss, type of hearing loss, state of the loss (i.e., temporary, permanent, fluctuating, or degenerative), emotional status, environmental factors, and familial factors all must be assessed to determine the possible impact a hearing loss has on an individual.

As with many disabilities and in many ethnic groups, certain terms connote negative images about that group. Within the past few years, the term *deaf* has become offensive to some people who have hearing impairments because of the derogatory images associated with the term *deaf and dumb.* Other people take great pride in the term *deaf* and strongly affiliate themselves with Deaf culture. Some of these people take offense if they are called *hearing impaired.* People with any type of hearing loss, mild to profound, should be referred to as having a hearing impairment or loss.

INCIDENCE

Approximately 24 million Americans have some degree of hearing loss. A hearing loss can range from mild to profound and is unique to each individual. Hearing impairments affect individuals of all ages and can occur at any point in time. Some people are born with a hearing loss. These people are referred to as having a **congenital** loss. Others lose their hearing as a result of an illness or injury. Hearing loss as part of the aging process is the most prevalent reason for an **acquired** loss. Half of all people older than 75 have some degree of hearing loss, and 80%–90% of all people older than 85 have a hearing loss.

IDENTIFYING HEARING LOSS

Hearing loss is discussed both in terms of the **degree** of loss and the **type** of loss. These two factors are determined through audiological testing. There are two types of testing that are usually performed in a routine hearing screening: **air conduction** and **bone conduction.**

Bridges Beyond Sound
© 1996 Corinne K. Jensema
Paul H. Brookes Publishing Co., Inc.

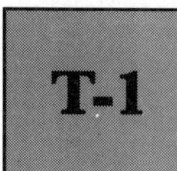

Air-Conduction Testing

Air-conduction testing is done using earphones, which are placed over a person's ears. Tones are then presented in one ear at a time. These tones vary in **frequencies** and **intensities.** Frequency is measured in Hertz (Hz) and intensity is measured in Decibels (dB). The intensity at which each frequency is heard is marked on a graph called an **audiogram.** Tones are normally presented at 250, 500, 1,000, 2,000, 4,000, and sometimes 8,000 Hz. The normal threshold of hearing (the lowest intensity at which a tone is heard) is between 0 dB and 15 dB. (Zero dB is not the absence of sound. It is the quietest sound that the average person with normal hearing can hear at that frequency.) The test usually begins by presenting a tone of 1,000 Hz at 0 dB. If the tone is not heard, the intensity is increased until either the person hears the tone or the intensity reaches 110 dB. Testing is typically not done beyond 110 dB because at that point the sound is so loud it can be felt. At the point at which the person heard the sound, a mark is placed on the audiogram indicating in which ear the tone was heard and that the tone was presented via air conduction. This is done for all of the frequencies listed above and for both ears.

Bone-Conduction Testing

Bone-conduction testing is used to determine whether a hearing loss detected in air-conduction testing resulted from conductive or sensorineural causes or a combination of the two. This type of testing uses the same methods as air conduction, but the tones are presented through a vibrator placed on the bone behind a person's ear. Tones are usually only presented at 500, 1,000, 2,000, and 4,000 Hz because of the limitations in bone-testing equipment and how the ear responds to this kind of testing. Again, the intensities at which the different frequency tones are detected are plotted on the audiogram.

DESCRIPTION OF HEARING LOSS

After audiological testing has been completed, the audiogram is read by the audiologist, who defines both the type and degree of the person's loss.

Type of Hearing Loss

The **type** of hearing loss refers to the physical cause of the loss. The results of the audiogram will indicate which part of the hearing mechanism has become damaged. Some hearing losses can be corrected by surgery or decreased in severity with the help of a hearing aid. However, not every person with a hearing loss can be helped by either of these methods. There are three main types of hearing loss: **conductive, sensorineural,** and **mixed.**

Conductive A conductive loss means that the loss is caused by anomalies or dysfunction of the outer or middle ear. In many cases, this type of loss can be surgically corrected. One characteristic of this type of loss is that the person may still be able to hear his or her own voice at a normal level but is unable to hear external sound. Ear infections and fluid in the middle ear can cause a temporary conductive hearing loss.

Sensorineural A sensorineural loss means that the hearing loss has been caused by dysfunction of the inner ear or auditory nerve. This type of hearing loss is permanent.

Bridges Beyond Sound
© 1996 Corinne K. Jensema
Paul H. Brookes Publishing Co., Inc.

With this type of loss, a person may not be able to hear his or her own voice or external sounds.

Mixed A mixed loss means that the hearing loss has both conductive and sensorineural components. This type of loss varies greatly from person to person. Some conductive components may be correctable by surgery; however, the sensorineural components would remain.

Degree of Hearing Loss

The degree (severity) of hearing loss refers to a person's hearing threshold. The hearing threshold is the quietest sound a person can hear at the frequencies measured by the audiogram. There are six categories of severity of loss: **normal, slight, mild, moderate, severe,** and **profound.**

Normal People with normal hearing can have a hearing threshold (i.e., loudness level) of 0 dB–15 dB. At this level, an individual can hear all speech sounds and will not experience any disabling effects.

Slight People with a slight hearing loss have a hearing threshold of 15 dB–25 dB. At this level, an individual can hear all vowel sounds but may not hear some unvoiced consonants, such as *f, t, p, k, ch, h,* and *s*. Some speech and language delay may be experienced by children who have this level of loss during the early developmental period.

Mild People with a mild hearing loss have a hearing threshold of 25 dB–40 dB. At this level, an individual can hear only some vowel sounds and loudly voiced consonants, such as *l, m,* and *n*. The effects of this kind of hearing loss may include articulation (i.e., speech) disorders, language delays, inattention, and auditory comprehension difficulties.

Moderate People with a moderate hearing loss have a hearing threshold of 40 dB–65 dB. At this level, an individual cannot hear most speech sounds at a normal conversational level. The effects of this kind of hearing loss may include articulation disorders, severe language delay, inattention, and learning difficulties.

Severe People with a severe hearing loss have a hearing threshold of 65 dB–95 dB. At this level, an individual can hear no speech sounds at a normal conversational level. The effects of this kind of hearing loss may include severe articulation disorders, severe language delay, learning difficulties, and inattention.

Profound People with a profound hearing loss have a hearing threshold of 95 dB or more. (The threshold of pain is 130 dB; any sound at this level is painful to a person with normal hearing.) At this level, an individual hears *no* speech sounds and few environmental sounds. The effects of this kind of hearing loss may include severe articulation impairments, severe language delay, learning difficulties, and inattention.

EFFECTS OF HEARING LOSS

Hearing impairments are very complex, and the types of difficulties people with hearing impairments encounter in communication are as complicated as the physical loss itself. The most important characteristic to remember is that the hearing loss diminishes a person's ability to understand spoken language. Many people who have hearing impairments cannot hear others speak or even hear their own voices. This characteristic alone seriously affects the language development of children who have a hearing loss.

Bridges Beyond Sound
© 1996 Corinne K. Jensema
Paul H. Brookes Publishing Co., Inc.

A hearing loss also affects each person's ability to learn language depending on several different factors. An infant with a hearing loss will experience more severe language impairments than an adult who acquires a hearing loss. The infant's language development can be significantly impaired by even a slight hearing loss, while the adult's language will not be seriously affected by the same slight loss.

The elements that determine the effects of a particular hearing loss include the nature and age of onset of the hearing loss, the emotional status of the person with a hearing loss, and any additional disability the person with a hearing loss might have.

The Nature of Hearing Loss

The nature of a hearing loss refers to the characteristics of the loss and the cause. A hearing loss can be **temporary, permanent, fluctuating,** or **degenerative.**

Temporary Temporary hearing losses can be acquired at any time and can last a day or several years depending on the cause. These hearing losses can be the result of trauma to the ear mechanism, illness, or serious chronic ear infections.

Permanent Permanent (lifelong) hearing losses are those with which some individuals are born and others acquire that remain with them throughout their lives. These hearing losses can be hereditary or the result of an illness or trauma to the hearing mechanism.

Fluctuating Fluctuating hearing losses change in severity from day to day. They can be acquired at any time. A person who has a fluctuating hearing loss will respond differently from day to day.

Degenerative Degenerative hearing losses are those whereby the severity of the loss increases over time. The change in hearing status can be very gradual, or significant changes can occur over a short period of time. This type of hearing loss can be hereditary or the result of an illness or trauma to the ear mechanism.

Age of Onset

The age of onset refers to when the hearing loss was incurred. There are three categories describing the age of onset: **congenital, acquired,** and **presbycusis.**

Congenital Congenital refers to a hearing loss that was present at birth and may be the result of hereditary factors, illness, or trauma. Individuals who have a congenital hearing loss experience more of the disabling effects of a hearing loss, regardless of the type or level, because the hearing loss is present while the child develops language.

Acquired An acquired hearing loss can occur or develop at any time during a person's life. Some individuals lose their hearing as young children, some as adolescents, and many as adults. This type of hearing loss can be the result of heredity, illness, or trauma. The effects of the hearing loss will vary greatly depending on the person's age, stage of development, and psychological status. In most cases, the younger a person who acquires a hearing loss is, the more difficulties he or she will experience.

Presbycusis Presbycusis is the term used to describe a hearing loss that occurs naturally as a person ages. This refers to a gradual loss that occurs after people reach approximately 60 years of age. The most important effects of this kind of hearing loss include acceptance and adjusting to the use of hearing aids.

Bridges Beyond Sound
© 1996 Corinne K. Jensema
Paul H. Brookes Publishing Co., Inc.

T-1

Emotional Status

The emotional status of an individual who has a hearing loss can greatly affect his or her ability to perform and reach his or her maximum potential. Each person who has a hearing loss handles the loss and its effects on his or her own life. A person who acquires a loss usually has a more difficult time accepting the circumstances than a person who was born with a hearing impairment. A hearing loss affects all aspects of a person's life. People who acquire a hearing loss may experience difficulty communicating with their families, gaining acceptance, continuing to function at their jobs, completing daily tasks without assistance, wearing and adjusting to hearing aids, and enjoying their usual forms of entertainment.

Additional Disabilities

A hearing loss may accompany one or many additional disabilities. The cause of the hearing loss may cause other disabilities as well. The presence of multiple disabilities may cause the effects of the disability to compound.

DEAF CULTURE

For centuries, people who are deaf have developed their own *deaf community*. This community has its own history and heritage just like any other ethnic group of people. Deaf community members have their own language, and they share many of the same experiences throughout their lives. Their heritage is passed down from deaf parents to their children and from one person who is deaf to another through deaf humor and signlore.

Deaf Humor

Deaf humor, an important aspect of Deaf culture, takes a look at the world from the point of view of a person who has a hearing impairment. People who are deaf laugh at themselves and the situations in which they find themselves in everyday life. Many jokes are visual plays on words, like verbal jokes play on words. A sign may be altered slightly to look like another sign, thus giving a sentence a different, funny meaning; or the sign may be made on a different part of the body to change the meaning. For example, if the sign for *weak* is made on the forehead instead of the opposite hand, it means *feeble-minded*. Deaf jokes are usually hard for people who can hear to understand.

Signlore

Signlore, another important part of Deaf culture, is a way of handing down stories, events, and finger games in sign language. These stories are not written, but passed on from one person who is deaf to another manually. Signlore and humor form common denominators for all people who are deaf, just as nursery rhymes and jokes do for people who can hear. People who are deaf feel very proud to be a part of the deaf community and Deaf culture.

Bridges Beyond Sound
© 1996 Corinne K. Jensema
Paul H. Brookes Publishing Co., Inc.

T-1

DEAF EDUCATION

Every parent who has a child with a hearing impairment has the same goal for his or her child. Parents want their children to learn to communicate and reach their highest potential. The educational methods they choose to help their children reach this goal vary.

Since the inception of education for the deaf, two opposing philosophies have existed—the oral (aural) method and the manual method. As of 1996, there are no effective assessment tools to determine at the time a hearing loss is diagnosed whether a child will be more successful in an oral or manual program. The family is given the task of choosing a method for their child.

Oral Method

The *oral (aural) method* of educating people who are deaf promotes teaching speechreading and oral speech to children with hearing impairments through the use of hearing aids and residual hearing training. One benefit of this method is that, if the training is successful, the child learns to understand and speak English. Knowing how to speak English allows a child an opportunity to function as independently as possible in the hearing world. In addition, an orally educated person often has more choices in higher education and employment.

Another benefit of this method is that family members do not have to learn a new form of communication. In the oral method, the family is taught strategies to encourage the child with a hearing impairment to pick up verbal language through speechreading and residual hearing training.

The success of the oral method varies greatly, however. If parents opt to have their child educated in the oral method, it is critical that the child's hearing loss is diagnosed as early as possible and the child is placed in an oral program. The longer a child develops without his or her hearing loss being diagnosed, the more language experiences he or she misses. The most critical language development period in a child's life is from birth to 4 years of age. Because many children's hearing impairments are not discovered until 2–3 years of age, several years of language learning and exposure have been lost. This delay often causes the child to perform at 2–3 years below the average child in his or her language and skill development throughout his or her education. This may place a child at a disadvantage for an oral program.

One of the major drawbacks to the oral method is that not all children are successful in developing oral and aural skills sufficient to communicate successfully with people who can hear. Depending on a variety of factors, a child's speech may not be intelligible and he or she may not become a proficient speechreader, which are two essential components of communicating with the hearing world. Even with disability awareness and teacher in-service programs (i.e., instruction provided to teachers by the school systems), children with hearing impairments who attend general classes often find that their peers and teachers do not relate well with them. An oral child may be the only child with a hearing loss in the school. In addition, students practiced in the oral method are discouraged from learning sign language during their education, leaving them unable to communicate manually with their peers who have been educated in the manual method.

Bridges Beyond Sound
© 1996 Corinne K. Jensema
Paul H. Brookes Publishing Co., Inc.

T-1

Another disadvantage arises when the oral method proves to be unsuccessful for a child. It is very difficult to change educational strategies midstream. For example, a child learning the oral method who is placed in a manual program will often find him- or herself without an effective communication system and may lose more language development time trying to learn sign language. Adults who adhere to the manual method often voice the opinion that the oral method isolates a person with a hearing impairment in both the hearing and deaf worlds. The person practiced in the oral method must try to integrate him- or herself into one or both of these worlds. For a child, this is a formidable task. The person educated through this method may not communicate effectively with people who can hear and if he or she does not know sign language, communicating with people educated in the manual method is nearly impossible. This can be devastating to a person's social-emotional growth and self-esteem. One solution to this problem is for people educated in the oral method to learn sign language as adults.

Manual Method

The *manual method* of education promotes teaching children with hearing impairments sign language. It also encourages the use of hearing aids if prescribed by an audiologist. The sign language most commonly used in the United States is American Sign Language (ASL). ASL is a true language, with its own grammar, syntax, and rules of use.

The major benefit of the manual method is that a child is given exposure to a language system that is accessible to him or her because it is visually based. This allows a child to learn language at a near typical rate, once exposed to sign language. Again, it is crucial that the child's hearing loss be diagnosed early and an appropriate educational setting be offered. It has been suggested that deaf children of deaf parents who communicate using sign language have the least difficulty with language development because they are exposed to sign language from birth (Jensema & Trybres, 1978). These children develop similarly to hearing children in a hearing family.

The manual method allows a child to be given all academic and social information through a communication mode that is not hampered by his or her hearing loss. This system also offers the opportunity for a child to become part of Deaf culture. An education system that promotes the use of ASL will usually provide students with an opportunity to share experiences associated with Deaf culture.

One limitation of the manual method is that ASL is a language different from English. ASL is a visually based language (i.e., communication is structured to be understandable as the eye sees it), whereas English is auditorially based and is structured to be understandable as the ear hears it. Often, people educated in the manual method do not read and write English well. This may lead to problems in higher education and in the workplace.

Another disadvantage of the manual method is that ASL is used by only a small segment of the population, those people with hearing impairments and hearing people who have learned to sign. People who use the manual method are limited in their ability to communicate with the hearing world and must often depend on a family member, friend, or professional sign language interpreter to communicate with hearing people. This may limit a person's independence.

Bridges Beyond Sound
© 1996 Corinne K. Jensema
Paul H. Brookes Publishing Co., Inc.

T-1

Finally, when a hearing family with a child who has a hearing impairment decides to educate the child using the manual method, the family members must also learn sign language in order to communicate effectively with the child. This can present problems because some people may have trouble learning sign language as quickly and as efficiently as the child with a hearing impairment. A vivid example of this problem was illustrated in the film, *Children of a Lesser God*, in which the main character, a deaf woman played by Marlee Matlin, discusses with her mother why their relationship has been so problematic over the years. The mother indicates that it was very difficult for her to learn to sign, whereas the daughter learned to sign quickly. The mother was frustrated and embarrassed that she could not communicate as well as her daughter, and this put a strain on their relationship from the time the daughter was a child.

Other deaf education strategies include **cued speech** and **total communication.** Cued speech was developed by Dr. Orin Cornett at Gallaudet University. This system is visually based and identifies all the sounds in the English language through the use of hand signals. This is not a language system in itself, but a strategy used in oral programs to assist children in learning to speechread and speaking verbal English.

Total communication is a philosophy that encourages the use of any and all communication methods that enable children with hearing impairments to communicate and receive communication. Typically, *simultaneous communication* (i.e., speech and a manual English method) is used on a conversational basis.

REFERENCES

Committee on Nomenclature, Conference of Executives of American Schools for the Deaf. (1938). *American Annals of the Deaf, 83,*1.

Federal Register. (1992, September 29). *57*(189), 44801.

Individuals with Disabilities Education Act (IDEA) of 1990, PL 101-476. (October 30, 1990). Title 20, U.S.C. 1400 et seq: *U.S. Statutes at Large, 104,* 1103–1151.

Jensema, C.J., & Trybres, R.J. (1978). *Communication patterns and education achievement of hearing impaired students.* Washington, DC: Gallaudet University.

Bridges Beyond Sound
© 1996 Corinne K. Jensema
Paul H. Brookes Publishing Co., Inc.

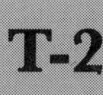

Questions Commonly Asked by Children About People Who Have Hearing Impairments

You may find that your students ask the following questions. Here are some answers to help you respond to them.

HOW DO I TALK TO PEOPLE WITH HEARING IMPAIRMENTS?

There are many ways to communicate with people who have hearing impairments. The following are some suggestions:

- Speak clearly and make sure the person who has a hearing impairment can see your face.
- Write down the message.
- Draw a picture.
- Point to what you are talking about.
- Gesture with your hands.
- Fingerspell your message.
- Use sign language.
- Use pantomime.
- Make sure a light source is on your face, not behind you.

WHY IS IT SOMETIMES HARD TO UNDERSTAND PEOPLE WHO ARE DEAF WHEN THEY TALK?

People who are deaf sound different because they cannot hear their own voices. If you cannot understand something a person who is deaf has said, ask him or her to say it again or write it down. Deaf people who use their voices encounter this every day and will not be offended. They have to practice rewording their messages so that they can be better understood. It is important to show that you are actively trying to understand.

CAN PEOPLE WHO ARE DEAF DRIVE CARS?

People who have hearing impairments are allowed to drive if they have drivers' licenses, just like everyone else. They may not be able to hear sirens and car horns, but they compensate for that by keeping very visually alert.

CAN PEOPLE WHO ARE DEAF LISTEN TO MUSIC?

Many people who have hearing impairments enjoy music. Some may be able to hear certain musical sounds; others enjoy the vibrations that music makes.

CAN PEOPLE WHO ARE DEAF DANCE?

Many people who are deaf enjoy dancing just as they enjoy music. Some people who have hearing impairments study dance as an art form. They appreciate the visual beauty of dance and have developed their own dance forms that incorporate sign language and poetry into movement. Sometimes people who have hearing impairments hold social dances where the music is loud enough to be heard or felt by everyone.

WHY DO PEOPLE WHO ARE DEAF SOMETIMES MAKE "FUNNY" SOUNDS?

Many people who have hearing impairments cannot hear their own voices. They cannot tell how loud or what pitch their voice is, or, more important, what kind of sound they are making. Many times when they are

Bridges Beyond Sound
© 1996 Corinne K. Jensema
Paul H. Brookes Publishing Co., Inc.

T-2

experiencing emotion or doing daily activities, they produce sounds of which they are unaware. Some examples include making unusual noises when they talk, speaking too loudly or softly, speaking in a strained pitch, or making smacking noises while eating.

CAN PEOPLE WHO ARE DEAF RIDE BICYCLES?

People who have hearing impairments can learn to ride bicycles just like everyone else. Their hearing impairments do not affect their ability to learn to ride bicycles. They must be cautious of traffic when riding just like anyone else, particularly because they cannot hear traffic noises. They can compensate for their hearing loss by using mirrors and staying very visually alert. Sometimes, the cause of a hearing impairment also causes a loss of balance because the mechanism for balance is located in the inner ear. People who have a hearing loss and also have no sense of balance must use their vision and sense of touch to compensate. They do this on bicycles as well.

HOW DO PEOPLE WHO ARE DEAF KNOW IF AN AMBULANCE IS COMING?

Each person who has a hearing impairment is different. Some people can still hear certain loud sounds, some may be able to hear the siren with their hearing aids, and others cannot hear anything at all but may see the flashing lights. Because many people who are deaf use lights for all kinds of alerting situations (e.g., telephone, doorbell), they are especially attuned to responding to light signals.

HOW DO PEOPLE WHO ARE DEAF KNOW IF THERE IS SOMEONE AT THE DOOR?

Each person who has a hearing impairment is different. Some may be able to hear a doorbell, but people who cannot may have visual *alerting systems* connected to their doorbells that flash lights when someone rings the doorbell. These lights are typically put in parts of the house where they can be readily seen and are not necessarily on the door itself.

HOW DO PEOPLE WHO ARE DEAF TALK ON THE TELEPHONE?

Again, each person who has a hearing impairment is different. Some just need a volume control button on their telephone to make it louder, others use hearing aids that have a telephone feature on them that helps the person hear on the telephone, and others use a telecommunication device for the deaf (TDD). The TDD is a machine connected to the telephone on which a person types. The person on the other end of the line also must have a TDD to receive the communication and respond back in the same way. The TDD is connected to the telephone through an acoustic coupler typically built on top of the TDD.

HOW DOES SOMEONE BECOME DEAF?

There are many different ways a person may lose his or her hearing. The most common causes are old age, heredity, and disease. Some people are born deaf. They may have become deaf because of an inherited syndrome, because their mother contracted or had a disease while they were in utero, or because of some developmental malformation or immaturity. Some people become deaf during the birthing process from lack of oxygen (i.e.,

Bridges Beyond Sound
© 1996 Corinne K. Jensema
Paul H. Brookes Publishing Co., Inc.

T-2

anoxia). Others lose their hearing at any time during their lives from such diseases as meningitis, high fevers, accidents or trauma (e.g., explosions, loud machinery, gunfire, brain trauma, rock music concerts), or the aging process.

ARE THEIR PARENTS DEAF?

Most children who are deaf have parents who can hear, and most parents who are deaf have children who can hear. Usually, only families that have *hereditary* deafness have several family members with hearing impairments. In these families, Deaf culture may be passed down from parent to child, rather than from peer to peer.

CAN PEOPLE WHO ARE DEAF HAVE BABIES?

People who are deaf can have children just like anyone else. Most people who are deaf have children who can hear.

CAN PEOPLE WHO ARE DEAF GET MARRIED?

Adults who have hearing impairments get married just like adults who can hear. Some marry other people who have hearing impairments, and others marry people who can hear. Marriages of people who both have a hearing impairment are most common among those who consider themselves culturally deaf.

DO PEOPLE WHO ARE DEAF GO TO SCHOOL?

Children with hearing impairments have a right to a free and appropriate public education just like other children. Some children who are deaf go to residential schools for the deaf where all of their special needs are addressed in one place and where almost everyone in the school knows sign language. Often, residential schools for the deaf help the children feel like a part of the deaf community and allow them to learn Deaf culture. Others are in classes specifically for the deaf in public schools or are included (full- or part-time) in general classes. Children with hearing impairments require special instructional materials, technologies, and methods to be successful.

CAN DEAF PEOPLE PLAY AND HAVE FUN?

Children who have hearing impairments like to play as much as children who can hear. They play the same games that hearing children play with the exception of games that depend totally on auditory cues, such as "Musical Chairs." Some games that depend on hearing can be adapted for children who are deaf. For instance, in "Musical Chairs," turning the lights on and off can be substituted for or used in conjunction with turning on and off the music. Children who are deaf, especially those who have loss of balance, may be averse to games where they are blindfolded, such as "Blind Man's Bluff" or "Pin the Tail on the Donkey."

Bridges Beyond Sound
© 1996 Corinne K. Jensema
Paul H. Brookes Publishing Co., Inc.

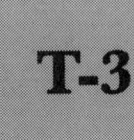

Glossary of Terminology Related to Hearing Loss and People Who Have Hearing Impairments

ACQUIRED HEARING LOSS — This type of loss can occur or develop at any time during a person's life. Some individuals lose their hearing as young children, some as adolescents, and many as adults. This type of hearing loss can be the result of heredity, illness, or trauma.

AGE OF ONSET — When a hearing loss is incurred.

AIR-CONDUCTION TESTING — A method of audiological testing whereby tones are presented to a person through earphones. This type of testing is routinely done to detect the presence of a hearing loss and its severity. Further testing must be done to determine the physical cause and type of loss.

ALERTING DEVICES — Devices used to inform people who have hearing impairments of events that people who can hear learn about through sound. An example would be a flashing light to tell them that the telephone is ringing. Most alerting devices for people who have hearing impairments use flashing lights or vibrators. Alerting devices are available for telephones, doorbells, alarm clocks, fire alarms, burglar alarms, and beepers.

AMERICAN SIGN LANGUAGE (ASL) — The only sign *language* indigenous to deaf people in the United States. This language involves hand, head, and upper body movements. It is not spoken or written.

AMPLIFIER — Any device that increases the loudness of a signal. People who have hearing impairments use many types of amplifiers, including hearing aids, telephone amplifiers, loop systems, and auditory trainers.

ANVIL — The second bone in the middle ear, also called the *incus*. This bone is connected on one end to the hammer and on the other end to the stirrup.

AUDIOGRAM — A graph that illustrates an individual's hearing loss. It indicates how much of a loss is present in each ear and what kind of loss is present. Often, an audiogram is interpreted by an audiologist to determine whether a person should use a hearing aid.

Bridges Beyond Sound
© 1996 Corinne K. Jensema
Paul H. Brookes Publishing Co., Inc.

T-3

BONE-CONDUCTION TESTING A method of audiological testing in which tones are presented to a person through a vibrator placed on the bone behind the ear. This method helps to determine if the hearing loss is caused by damage to the inner ear or auditory nerve.

CLOSED CAPTIONING The system that enables people with hearing impairments to watch and understand television, films, and videotapes through subtitles. In order to see subtitles or closed captioning, the viewer must have a device called a *decoder* attached to or built into his or her television that interprets the coded words that appear on the television screen. The viewer can identify programs and films that are closed captioned by the symbol CC. All televisions with screens 13 inches or greater built after July 1993 have closed-captioning capabilities.

COCHLEA The innermost portion of the ear. It is a coiled mechanism that is filled with fluid. When the ear transmits sound waves, the fluid in the cochlea moves. This fluid then moves over cilia (i.e., hairs) that wave back and forth with the movement of the fluid. These hairs have nerves attached to them and when moved send electrical signals to the brain.

CONDUCTIVE HEARING LOSS A hearing loss that is caused by anomalies or dysfunction of the outer or middle ear.

CONGENITAL HEARING LOSS A hearing loss that was present at birth and may be the result of hereditary factors, illness, or trauma.

CUED SPEECH This communication system is visually based and identifies all the sounds in the English language through the use of hand signals. This is not a language system in itself, but a strategy used in oral programs to assist children to learn to speechread and speak English.

DEAF Deaf is defined by the Committee on Nomenclature, Conference of Executives of American Schools for the Deaf, as a condition wherein a hearing loss is so severe that the person has an impairment in processing linguistic information through hearing, with or without amplification.

DEAF CULTURE This culture shares a common language, American Sign Language (ASL), life experiences, storytelling, humor, and history. Many, but not all, people

Bridges Beyond Sound
© 1996 Corinne K. Jensema
Paul H. Brookes Publishing Co., Inc.

T-3

who are deaf consider themselves to be members of this culture. It can be handed down from a parent who is deaf to a child who is deaf or from a peer who is deaf to another peer.

DECIBEL (dB) A unit of loudness. Decibels (dB) are used to measure the level of sound. Hearing loss is described in terms of the decibel level to which sound must be amplified in order for a particular person to hear it. Audiograms measure hearing loss in terms of decibels.

DECODER A device that makes subtitles or closed captions appear on a television screen so that a person has a written account of the dialogue and other auditory information aired. The device is attached to or built into the television set.

DEGENERATIVE HEARING LOSS A hearing loss whereby the severity of the loss increases over time. The change in hearing status can be very gradual, or significant changes can occur over a short period of time. This type of hearing loss can be caused by hereditary factors or as a result of illness or trauma to the ear mechanism.

EAR CANAL The tube that leads inside the ear from the pinna. This is where earwax is found.

EARDRUM A membrane that stretches across the ear canal at its furthest point inside the head. The eardrum vibrates when sound waves hit it. The eardrum is also called the *tympanic membrane.*

EARMOLD A flexible rubber or acrylic mold made to fit the outer ear of an individual hearing aid owner.

EUSTACHIAN TUBE A ventilation tube that runs from the middle ear to the oral cavity. The eustachian tube is responsible for making ears pop and for draining fluid out of the ear when a person has an ear infection.

FINGERSPELLING Manual representations of the alphabet.

Bridges Beyond Sound
© 1996 Corinne K. Jensema
Paul H. Brookes Publishing Co., Inc.

T-3

FLUCTUATING HEARING LOSS A hearing loss that can change in severity from day to day.

HAMMER The first of the three bones inside the middle ear (also called the *malleus*). This bone is connected on one end to the eardrum and to the anvil (incus) on the other end.

HEARING AIDS Devices that amplify sound and are used by some people who have hearing impairments to assist them in identifying environmental sounds and some speech. Not all people who have hearing impairments can use a hearing aid.

HEARING THRESHOLD The quietest sound a person can hear at the frequencies measured by an audiogram. The hearing threshold is used to describe the severity of a hearing loss.

HEREDITARY DEAFNESS A hearing loss that is the result of hereditary factors rather than all other causes of hearing impairment. This type of hearing impairment is passed from one generation to the next by genetic information. Each family member's hearing loss will be unique. Some may be born deaf, some may lose their hearing as children, and some may lose their hearing as adults. In addition, not every generation will produce family members with hearing losses. This type of hereditary trait can skip several generations.

HERTZ (Hz) How sound frequency (i.e., pitch) is measured. Hearing is tested at various frequencies measured in Hertz (Hz). An audiogram illustrates the different Hertz at which hearing is tested.

INCLUSION The philosophy and practice of using teaching strategies that allow for a student with a disability to participate effectively in general education. The rationale for this practice is that children with special needs must be integrated with their peers who do not have disabilities in order to develop appropriate social relationships and become experienced with the world outside the classroom. The practice has benefits for the students without disabilities as well.

INTERPRETER A person who is trained and certified as a sign language or oral interpreter. Interpreters translate for people who have hearing impairments in many

Bridges Beyond Sound
© 1996 Corinne K. Jensema
Paul H. Brookes Publishing Co., Inc.

T-3

different settings in which they need to communicate with people who can hear and in which it is imperative that they communicate effectively. They are used in classrooms, at work, at meetings, at religious services, and at special events. When a person who can hear is communicating with a person who has a hearing impairment through an interpreter, the hearing person should speak directly to the person with the hearing impairment rather than with the interpreter.

MANUAL METHOD This method promotes teaching children with hearing impairments to communicate through sign language.

MILD HEARING LOSS A hearing threshold of 25 dB–40 dB. At this level an individual can hear only some vowel sounds and loudly voiced consonants, such as *l, m,* and *n.*

MIXED HEARING LOSS A hearing loss that has both conductive and sensorineural components.

MODERATE HEARING LOSS A hearing threshold of 40 dB–65 dB. At this level, an individual cannot hear most speech sounds at a normal conversational level.

NORMAL HEARING A hearing threshold of 0 dB–15 dB.

OPEN CAPTIONING This type of television captioning does not require the use of a decoder in order to view the subtitles. The captions appear at all times and can be viewed by anyone. Open captioning is often seen on news broadcasts or at public events.

ORAL METHOD This method promotes teaching speechreading and oral speech to children with hearing impairments through associated strategies, hearing aids, and training of residual hearing.

PERMANENT HEARING LOSS A hearing loss that some individuals are born with and others acquire that remains with them throughout their lives. A permanent hearing loss can be hereditary or the result of illness or trauma to the hearing mechanism.

PIDGIN SIGN ENGLISH (PSE) A hybrid of English and American Sign Language that combines features of both and contains many of the characteristics of other pidgin languages.

Bridges Beyond Sound
© 1996 Corinne K. Jensema
Paul H. Brookes Publishing Co., Inc.

T-3

PINNA
The external portion of the ear. The function of the pinna is to direct sound waves into the ear canal.

PRESBYCUSIS
The term used to describe a hearing loss that occurs naturally as a person ages. This refers to a gradual loss that occurs after people reach approximately 60 years of age.

PROFOUND HEARING LOSS
A hearing threshold of 95 dB and above. At this level, an individual hears no speech sounds and few environmental sounds.

RESIDUAL HEARING
This term refers to the degree of hearing a person with a hearing loss has remaining. For example, if a person has a 50 dB loss, he or she can still hear sounds at 50 dB and higher. A hearing aid can be used to amplify sound to a person's residual hearing level. However, this does not mean that the person can understand spoken language. The ability to discriminate sounds and understand language is also determined by the type of loss a person has.

SENSORINEURAL HEARING LOSS
A hearing loss that is caused by dysfunction of the inner ear or auditory nerve.

SEVERE HEARING LOSS
A hearing threshold of 65 dB–95 dB. At this level, an individual can hear *no* speech sounds at a normal conversational level.

SIGNED EXACT ENGLISH (SEE)
A manual form of English. It is a signed system versus a true language. Some of the vocabulary used is adapted from American Sign Language; however, the structure is English, not American Sign Language. The system was developed with the intent to assist children with hearing impairments while being taught manually to learn English. SEE is much easier for people who can hear to learn because it follows English word order and structure.

SIGNLORE
A way of handing down stories, events, and finger games in sign language. These stories are not written, but passed on from one deaf person to another manually.

SLIGHT HEARING LOSS
A hearing threshold of 15 dB–25 dB. At this level, an individual can hear all vowel sounds but may not hear some unvoiced consonants, such as *f, t, p, k, ch, h,* and *s.*

Bridges Beyond Sound
© 1996 Corinne K. Jensema
Paul H. Brookes Publishing Co., Inc.

T-3

SPEECHREADING — A technique used by some people with hearing impairments to understand spoken language by visually analyzing mouth and other facial movements. It also includes learning to read a situation for environmental cues and body language. This technique is extremely difficult to master and is dependent on many factors, including the speaker's accent, mouth movement, lighting, position, and whether there is a facial obstruction like a beard or moustache.

STIRRUP — The third and last bone in the middle ear (also called the *stapes*). This bone is connected to the anvil (incus) on one end and to a membrane called the *round window* on the other.

TELECOMMUNICATION DEVICE FOR THE DEAF (TDD) — A machine that was developed to allow people with hearing impairments to use the telephone. TDDs connect to the telephone receiver and make it possible for a person to use a keyboard to type to another party who has a TDD. TDDs may also be referred to as *TTYs* (i.e., teletypewriters) or *TTs* (i.e., text telephones).

TEMPORARY HEARING LOSS — A hearing loss that can be acquired at any time and can last anywhere from a day to several years, depending on the cause. A temporary hearing loss can be the result of trauma to the ear mechanism, illness, or serious chronic ear infections.

TOTAL COMMUNICATION — A philosophy that promotes using any communication method that enables a child with a hearing impairment to communicate and receive communication. Typically, both speech and manual English are used simultaneously in casual conversation and during instruction.

Bridges Beyond Sound
© 1996 Corinne K. Jensema
Paul H. Brookes Publishing Co., Inc.

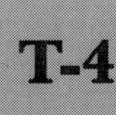

How to Use a TDD (TTY or TT)

RECEIVING A CALL

The following are instructions for receiving a call on a TDD:

1. TDD calls can be identified by one of the following:
   - An electronic beeping sound
   - Silence
   - A computerized voice announcing that a person who is using a TDD is calling
2. When a call is received and determined to be a TDD call, turn on the TDD and place the telephone receiver in the cups on top of the TDD, using the diagram on the TDD as a guide. If your TDD has a direct connect feature, you will not have to place the telephone receiver on top of the TDD.
3. Answer the call by typing "Hello," your name, and then GA. GA stands for *go ahead*, which tells the other person that it is his or her turn to type.
4. Wait for the caller's message and GA (your cue to respond).
5. Proceed with the call as you would a call from a hearing person, typing your responses to the caller. Remember to type GA when you want the caller to respond.
6. If all or part of the caller's message is garbled, request that the message be repeated. This is a common occurrence on TDD calls.
7. When you are finished with your side of the conversation, type your closing remarks followed by GASK, GA or SK, or GA to SK. This notifies the caller that you are ready to end the conversation. SK stands for *stop keying.*
8. The caller will make closing statements and type SKSK.
9. Hang up the telephone and turn off the TDD.

MAKING A CALL

The following are instructions for making a call on a TDD:

1. Turn on the TDD and place the telephone receiver in the cups on top of the TDD, using the diagram on the TDD as a guide. If your TDD has a direct connect feature, simply dial the telephone number from the TDD. Check the instruction manual for instructions on your specific machine.
2. Dial the telephone number of the person you are calling. The *signal light* on the TDD will flash as the telephone rings.
3. When the telephone is answered, the signal light will remain solidly lit. Press the space bar or some of the letter keys to let the person know you are calling on a TDD. If there is a hearing person on the other end, he or she will hear "tweedling" sounds.
4. The person you are calling may answer directly with a TDD. Monitor the message display for a response to your call.
5. Proceed with the call as described above, remembering to type GA to let the other party know to go ahead and SK when you are ready to stop keying.

Bridges Beyond Sound
© 1996 Corinne K. Jensema
Paul H. Brookes Publishing Co., Inc.

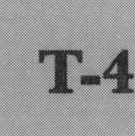

TROUBLESHOOTING TRANSMISSION PROBLEMS

TDD calls can become garbled because of weather conditions, telephone line interference, or external noise. If you are having problems with your TDD, the procedures below may help you correct the problem.

No Message Displayed

- Check the cable connections.
- Make sure the TDD is plugged in and the on/off switch is on.
- If the TDD is directly connected to the telephone line, make sure the telephone line is plugged securely into the TDD and into the telephone jack.
- If the TDD is powered by batteries, check to see if they are weak.

Garbled Message

- It is important to note that if you are receiving a garbled message, the other party may or may not be receiving one from you.
- Check that the telephone receiver fits snugly in the cups on top of the TDD, if appropriate. Otherwise, make sure that the telephone cord is plugged securely into the back of the TDD and into the telephone jack.
- Turn the TDD off and back on again. This will *not* disconnect your call and may improve the quality of the transmission.
- Ask the other person to type more slowly.
- If you have another TDD, try using it.
- Tell the caller that the message is garbled, and ask him or her to repeat the message and/or check his or her TDD.

TDD ETIQUETTE

Abbreviations are often used in TDD conversations to speed up communication. Some common abbreviations follow:

ASAP	As soon as possible
B4	Before
CUD	Could
CUZ	Because
GA	Go ahead

Bridges Beyond Sound
© 1996 Corinne K. Jensema
Paul H. Brookes Publishing Co., Inc.

T-4

HD	Hold
MTG	Meeting
NBR	Number
NP	No problem
OIC	Oh, I see
OK	Okay, all right
PH NBR	Telephone number
PLS	Please
Q	? (other punctuation is usually omitted in TDD conversations)
R	Are
SHUD	Should
SK	Stop keying
THX	Thanks
TMW	Tomorrow
U	You
UR	Your
WUD	Would
XXX	Error or mistake in typing

Bridges Beyond Sound
© 1996 Corinne K. Jensema
Paul H. Brookes Publishing Co., Inc.

T-4

- If you are sharing important information, such as telephone numbers, dates, or addresses, it is a good idea to repeat the information you have received to be sure there are no mistakes.
- Handling interruptions requires different strategies when using a TDD. Because you are communicating electronically, you cannot type at the same time the other person is typing. This will result in a garbled message. Interruptions should occur only for emergency reasons. To interrupt, hit the space bar several times or the letter X several times. If you need to leave the telephone, type PLS HD. When you can return to the telephone, explain to the other person what happened and why you asked him or her to hold.

Bridges Beyond Sound
© 1996 Corinne K. Jensema
Paul H. Brookes Publishing Co., Inc.

T-5

INTERPRETERS FOR PEOPLE WITH HEARING IMPAIRMENTS

Interpreters are used to assist in the communication between people with and without hearing impairments. Interpreters are professionals, and many have completed an accredited program of study and are members of the Registry of Interpreters for the Deaf (RID). RID provides testing and certification for interpreters and has established a Code of Ethics for professional interpreters.

Interpreters are used any time two or more people need to communicate with others or with each other, but they have different forms of communicating. PL 101-336, the Americans with Disabilities Act (ADA) of 1990, requires that any government-sponsored event (including school) open to the public provide sign language interpreting services for any people with hearing impairments who may attend. Interpreters are seen in virtually every setting—from schools, churches, synagogues, and hospitals to theaters and public meetings.

There are several different types of interpreters. **Oral interpreters** verbally repeat all the conversation for the person with a hearing loss, using speechreading techniques to ensure that the person understands the message. He or she may also repeat what the person with a hearing impairment says to ensure that his or her message is understood as well. **Sign interpreters** use American Sign Language (ASL), Pidgin Signed English (PSE), or Manually Coded English (MCE) to interpret spoken English into sign for the person with a hearing impairment and sign into spoken English for the hearing person. Although ASL is a true language with its own grammar and syntax, PSE and MCE are ways of representing English through signs. The sign system used depends on the person's individual needs.

An alternative technique for interpreting information is **notetaking.** When a person with a hearing impairment is in an audience in which information is being verbally transmitted, a notetaker writes down all the important components of a message. This allows the person with a hearing impairment to maintain eye contact with the speaker and participate in the activity without having to spend time writing down the important elements of the message.

In the classroom, interpreters are used when a student with a hearing impairment is included in a general education class or attends a function (e.g., assembly) that is primarily attended by hearing people. An interpreter is also used because a student who is deaf may not be able to communicate effectively with his or her peers or teacher. The interpreter sits in a strategic location and interprets all conversation that occurs in the class. This includes teacher instructions, student responses, class participation, peer-to-peer conversations, and general conversation. The interpreter is *not* a teacher or classroom aide. His or her function is to provide the student with all the same information that is available to the hearing students.

Teachers should follow the guidelines below when using an interpreter. They are applicable when communicating one-to-one with a student. In a lecture situation, they can be modified to provide the best possible communication situation for the student.

1. **Stand or sit next to the interpreter.**
   It is important to remember to sit or stand next to the interpreter, when possible, so that you can look and talk to the student, not the interpreter. This also enables the student to maintain visual contact with you and the interpreter simultaneously.

Bridges Beyond Sound
© 1996 Corinne K. Jensema
Paul H. Brookes Publishing Co., Inc.

T-5

2. **Place graphics or models near you and the interpreter.**
   Again, this is to ensure that the student can look at the speaker, interpreter, and the graphics without having to turn his or her head from one side to the other and perhaps miss important information being communicated through the interpreter while looking at the visual aid.
3. **Talk at a normal rate.**
   The interpreter has been trained to interpret messages at a normal conversational pace. There is no need, unless asked, to slow your speech for the interpreter.
4. **Maintain eye contact with the student.**
   You are communicating with the student, not the interpreter. It is considered rude to talk directly to the interpreter and not include the student in the conversation.
5. **Address your communication to the student, not the interpreter.**
   As stated above, you are communicating with the student. Speak directly to him or her. Do not say, "Tell him to get out his book"; rather, address the student directly, as in "David, get out your book."
6. **Allow time for the student to ask and respond to questions.**
   When using an interpreter, the conversation proceeds more slowly than when two people can communicate directly with each other. Make sure you allow enough time for the interpreter to communicate your message to the student, for the student to respond, and for the interpreter to voice the response to you.

REFERENCES

Americans with Disabilities Act (ADA) of 1990, PL 101-336. (July 26, 1990). Title 42, U.S.C. 12101 et seq: *U.S. Statutes at Large, 104,* 327–378.

Bridges Beyond Sound
© 1996 Corinne K. Jensema
Paul H. Brookes Publishing Co., Inc.

T-6

SELECTED READINGS AND VIDEOTAPES ABOUT DEAFNESS AND PEOPLE WHO ARE DEAF

Below is a list of select published materials relating to deafness and deaf education. For additional publications, you are encouraged to contact the National Information Center on Deafness (NICD) at Gallaudet University in Washington, D.C., and request copies of the annotated bibliography, *Have You Ever Wondered About Hearing Loss and Deafness?* They may be reached by calling (202) 651-5051 or writing to NICD at 800 Florida Avenue, NE, Washington, D.C., 20002. They are also an excellent resource for fact sheets and informative brochures on all topics related to deafness. Most of these resources are free or can be purchased at a very low cost.

BIOGRAPHIES ON DEAF PEOPLE

Albronda, M. (1980). *Douglas Tilden: Portrait of a deaf sculptor.* Silver Spring, MD: T.J. Publishers.
Berg, O.B. (1989). *Thomas Gallaudet: Apostle to the deaf.* New York: St. Ann's Church for the Deaf.
Bessone, L.T. (1987, May 25). He didn't hear the roar. *Sports Illustrated, 66*(21), 20.
Bowe, F. (1973). *I'm deaf too: Twelve deaf Americans.* Silver Spring, MD: National Association of the Deaf.
Braddock, G.C. (1975). *Notable deaf persons.* Washington, DC: Gallaudet University Alumni Association.
Bragg, B. (1989). *Lessons in laughter: The autobiography of a deaf actor.* Washington, DC: Gallaudet University Press.
Bruce, R. (1973). *Alexander Graham Bell and the conquest of solitude.* Boston: Little, Brown.
Ferrigno, L. (1982). *The incredible Lou Ferrigno: His story.* New York: Simon & Schuster.
Hairston, E., & Smith, L. (1983). *Black and deaf in America: Are we that different?* Silver Spring, MD: T.J. Publishers.
Holcomb, M. (1989). *Deaf women: A parade through the decade.* Berkeley, CA: Dawn Sign Press.
Huston, C. (1973). *Deaf Smith, incredible Texan spy.* Waco, TX: Texian Press.
Jacobs, L.M. (1989). *A deaf adult speaks out.* Washington, DC: Gallaudet University Press.
Lane, H. (1984). *When the mind hears: A history of the deaf.* New York: Random House.
Luterman, D. (1987). *Deafness in the family.* San Diego, CA: College-Hill Press.
Marek, G.R. (1969). *Beethoven: Biography of a genius.* New York: Funk & Wagnalls.
Panara, R. (1983). *Great deaf Americans.* Silver Spring, MD: T.J. Publishers.
Quinn, E., & Owens, M. (1984). *Listen to me: The story of Elizabeth Quinn.* London: M. Joseph.
Schein, J.D. (1981). *A rose for tomorrow: Biography of Frederick C. Schreiber.* Silver Spring, MD: National Association of the Deaf.
Schuchman, J. (1988). *Hollywood speaks: Deafness and the film entertainment industry.* Urbana: University of Illinois Press.
Shepard, J. (Director/Producer), & Panara, J. (Narrator). (1980). *Famous deaf Americans: A videotaped program in two parts* [Videotape]. New York: National Technical Institute for the Deaf.
Spradley, T.S. (1978). *Deaf like me.* New York: Random House.

DEAF EDUCATION

Aiello, B. (1981). *The hearing impaired child in the regular class.* Washington, DC: AFT Teacher's Network for Education of the Handicapped.
Bender, R.E. (1981). *The conquest of deafness: A history of the long struggle to make possible normal living to those handicapped by lack of normal hearing.* Danville, IL: Interstate Printers & Publishers.
Bookbinder, S. (1978). *Mainstreaming: What every child needs to know about disabilities: The Meeting Street School curriculum for grades 1–4.* Boston: Exceptional Parent Press.
Bowe, F. (1991). *Approaching equality: Education of the deaf.* Silver Spring, MD: T.J. Publishers.
Davis, J. (1990). *Our forgotten children: Hard of hearing pupils in the schools.* Bethesda, MD: Self Help for Hard of Hearing People.
Fay, E.A. (1983). *Histories of American schools for the deaf.* Washington, DC: The Volta Bureau.
Griffith, A., & Scott, D. (Eds.). (1985). *Looking back—looking forward: Living with deafness.* Toronto, Ontario, Canada: Canadian Hearing Society.

Bridges Beyond Sound
© 1996 Corinne K. Jensema
Paul H. Brookes Publishing Co., Inc.

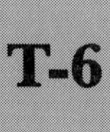

Higgins, P.C. (1990). *The challenge of educating together deaf and hearing youth: Making mainstreaming work.* Springfield, IL: Charles C Thomas.
Katz, L. (1974). *The deaf child in the public schools: A handbook for parents of deaf children.* Danville, IL: Interstate Printers & Publishers.
Lane, H. (Ed.). (1984). *The deaf experience: Classics in language and education.* Cambridge, MA: Harvard University Press.
Laporta, R.A. (1978). *Mainstreaming preschoolers: Children with hearing impairment. A guide for teachers, parents, and others who work with hearing impaired preschoolers.* Washington, DC: U.S. Government Printing Office.
Moores, D.F. (1987). *Educating the deaf: Psychology, principles, and practices.* Boston: Houghton Mifflin.
Nussbaum, D. (1988). *There's a hearing impaired child in my class: A learning packet about hearing loss for public school teachers.* Washington, DC: Gallaudet University Pre-College Programs.
Ogden, P.W. (1982). *The silent garden: Understanding the hearing-impaired child.* New York: St. Martin's Press.
Simmons-Martin, A. (1975). *Chats with Johnny's parents.* Washington, DC: Alexander Graham Bell Association for the Deaf.
Truax, R., & Shultz, J. (Eds.). (1983). *Learning to communicate: Implications for the hearing impaired.* Washington, DC: Alexander Graham Bell Association for the Deaf.
Winefield, R. (1987). *Never the twain shall meet: Bell, Gallaudet, and the communications debate.* Washington, DC: Gallaudet University Press.

SIGN LANGUAGE

Baker, C., & Padden, C. (1978). Focusing on the nonmanual components of American Sign Language. In P. Siple (Ed.), *Understanding language through sign language research.* New York: Academic Press.
Bornstein, H. (1973, June). A description of some current sign systems designed to represent English. *American Annals of the Deaf, 118,* 454–463.
Cokely, D. (1980). *American Sign Language: A teacher's resource text on curriculum, methods, and evaluation.* Silver Spring, MD: T.J. Publishers.
Cokely, D., & Ness, V. (Producers & Directors). (1992). *Working with a sign language interpreter* [Videotape]. Burtonsville, MD: Sign Media.
Costello, E. (1983). *Signing: How to speak with your hands.* New York: Bantam Books.
Dicker, L. (1981). *Facilitating manual communication for interpreters, students, and teachers.* Silver Spring, MD: Registry of Interpreters for the Deaf, Inc.
Evans, L. (1982). *Total communication: Structure and strategy.* Washington, DC: Gallaudet University Press.
Fant, L.J. (1972). *An introduction to American Sign Language.* Silver Spring, MD: National Association of the Deaf.
Grier, B. (Producer). (1989). *Communicating with the hearing impaired: An introductory course in American Sign Language* [Videotape]. Princeton, NJ: Films for the Humanities.
Guillory, L. (1974). *Expressive and receptive fingerspelling for hearing adults.* Baton Rouge, LA: Claitor's Publishing Division.
Gustason, G., Pfetzing, D., & Zawolkow, E. (1980). *Signing exact English.* Rossmoor, CA: Modern Signs Press.
Hoemann, H. (1978). *Communicating with deaf people: A resource manual for teachers and students of American Sign Language.* Baltimore: University Park Press.
Neisser, A. (1983). *The other side of silence: Sign language and the deaf community in America.* New York: Alfred A. Knopf.
Newell, W. (1983). *Basic sign communication.* Silver Spring, MD: National Association of the Deaf.
Parker, D. (Producer). (1990). *The sign for friends* [Videotape]. Pittsburgh, PA: Yellin Tabor Visual Productions.
Riekehof, L.L. (1978). *The joy of signing.* Springfield, MO: Gospel Publishing House.
Shroyer, S.P. (1988). *Secret signing: Grades 1–3.* Greensboro, NC: Sugar Sign Press.

DEAF CULTURE AND ENTERTAINMENT

Beinvenu, M.J., & Colonomus, B. (Writers). (1985). *Introduction to American Deaf culture: Rules of social interaction* [Videotape]. Burtonsville, MD: Sign Media.

Bridges Beyond Sound
© 1996 Corinne K. Jensema
Paul H. Brookes Publishing Co., Inc.

T-6

Benderly, B.L. (1980). *Dancing without music: Deafness in America.* Garden City, NY: Anchor Press/Doubleday.
Gannon, J. (1981). *Deaf heritage: A narrative history of deaf America.* Silver Spring, MD: National Association of the Deaf.
Gannon, J. (1989). *The week the world heard Gallaudet.* Washington, DC: Gallaudet University Press.
Glick, F.P. (1982). *Breaking silence: A family grows with deafness.* Scottsdale, PA: Herald Press.
Harris, G.A. (1983). *Broken ears, wounded hearts.* Washington, DC: Gallaudet University Press.
Holcomb, R.K. (1977). *Hazards of deafness.* Northridge, CA: Joyce Media.
Lane, L.G., & Pittle, I.B. (Eds.). (1981). *A handful of stories: Thirty-seven stories by deaf storytellers.* Washington, DC: Gallaudet University, Division of Public Services.
Mindel, E., & Vernon, M. (Eds.). (1987). *They grow in silence: Understanding deaf children and adults.* Boston: College-Hill Press.
Moore, M.S. (1993). *For hearing people only: Answers to some of the most commonly asked questions about the deaf community, its culture, and the "deaf reality."* Rochester, NY: Deaf Life Press.
National Association for Hearing and Speech Action. (1986). *Directory of assistive listening devices.* Rockville, MD: Author.
Olsen, G. (Ed.). (1987). *Kaleidoscope of deaf America.* Silver Spring, MD: National Association of the Deaf.
Padden, C. (1988). *Deaf in America: Voices from a culture.* Cambridge, MA: Harvard University Press.
Sacks, O. (1989). *Seeing voices: A journey into the world of the deaf.* Berkeley: University of California Press.
Steward, D.A. (1991). *Deaf sport: The impact of sports within the deaf community.* Washington, DC: Gallaudet University Press.
Stoker, R.G., & Spear, J.H. (Eds.). (1984, September). Hearing-impaired perspectives on living in the mainstream. *The Volta Review, 86*(5).
Trychin, S. (Author). (1987). *Did I do that?* [Videotape]. Washington, DC: Gallaudet University Press.
Van Cleve, J. (Ed.). (1987). *Gallaudet encyclopedia of deaf people and deafness.* New York: McGraw-Hill.
Van Cleve, J. (1989). *A place of their own: Creating the deaf community in America.* Washington, DC: Gallaudet University Press.
Wilcox, S. (1989). *American deaf culture: An anthology.* Silver Spring, MD: Linstock Press.

ASSISTIVE TECHNOLOGIES

Graham, B. (1978). *One thing led to the next: The real history of TTYs.* Evanston, IL: Mosquito Publishers.
Rosenthal, R. (1978). *The hearing loss handbook.* New York: Schocken Books.

Bridges Beyond Sound
© 1996 Corinne K. Jensema
Paul H. Brookes Publishing Co., Inc.

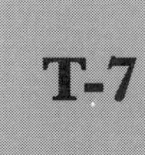

STATE ORGANIZATIONS OF AND FOR THE DEAF

Contact your state organization for the deaf and request that a representative come to your school to speak to students about deafness and Deaf culture. These organizations are also excellent resources for suggestions about field trips, speakers, and other activities on deaf awareness.

ALABAMA

Alabama State Association of the Deaf
16217 Highway 55
Sterett, AL 35147
(205) 672-8060 TDD

ALASKA

Alaska Association of the Deaf
1345 Rudakof Circle, #107
Anchorage, AK 99508
(907) 333-7545 TDD

ARIZONA

Arizona Association of the Deaf
8336 El Sells Drive
Scottsdale, AZ 85251
(602) 946-7009 TDD

ARKANSAS

Arkansas Association of the Deaf
9005 Lew Drive
Little Rock, AR 72209
(501) 565-4374 TDD

CALIFORNIA

California Association of the Deaf
38181 Hastings Court
Fremont, CA 94536
(510) 888-9521 TDD

COLORADO

Colorado Association of the Deaf
c/o Vedtiz Office
2785 North Speer Boulevard, #308
Denver, CO 80227
(303) 986-3583 TDD

CONNECTICUT

Greater Bridgeport Association of the Deaf
160 Taft Avenue
Bridgeport, CT 06606
(203) 367-7175 V/TDD

DELAWARE

Delaware Association of the Deaf
Post Office Box 8973
Newark, DE 19714

FLORIDA

Broward City Association of the Deaf
362 West Sample Road
Pompono Beach, FL 33064
(305) 784-0042 TDD

GEORGIA

Georgia Association of the Deaf
1104 Riverbend Drive
Dalton, GA 30720
(706) 278-0914 TDD

HAWAII

Aloha Association of the Deaf
1221 Victoria Street, #1405
Honolulu, HI 96814
(808) 524-4200 TDD

ILLINOIS

National Fraternal Society of the Deaf
1300 West Northwest Highway
Mt. Prospect, IL 60056
(708) 392-1409 TDD

Bridges Beyond Sound
© 1996 Corinne K. Jensema
Paul H. Brookes Publishing Co., Inc.

T-7

INDIANA

Indiana Association of the Deaf
445 North Penn Street, #804
Indianapolis, IN 46204
(317) 636-DEAF

IOWA

Iowa Association of the Deaf
Post Office Box 1
Council Bluffs, IA 51503
(712) 366-6006 TDD

KANSAS

Kansas Association of the Deaf
719 North Singletree
Olathe, KS 66061
(913) 791-0511 TDD

KENTUCKY

Louisville Association of the Deaf
2622 South 3rd Street
Louisville, KY 40208
(502) 778-4141 TDD

LOUISIANA

Louisiana Association of the Deaf
4864 Constitution Avenue, #2B
Baton Rouge, LA 70808
(504) 923-1266 V/TDD

MAINE

Self Help For Hard of Hearing People
243 Buck Street, #1
Bangor, ME 04401
(207) 947-4065 TDD

MARYLAND

Metro Washington Association of the Deaf
814 Thayer Avenue
Silver Spring, MD 20910
(301) 585-9084 TDD

MASSACHUSETTS

Massachusetts Association of the Deaf
11 Starbird Street, #3
Malden, MA 02148
(617) 322-1717 TDD

MICHIGAN

Michigan Association of the Deaf
724 Abbott Road
East Lansing, MI 48823
(517) 377-1649 TDD

MINNESOTA

Minnesota Association of the Deaf
804 6th Avenue, SW
Faribault, MN 55021
(612) 221-1337 V/TDD

MISSISSIPPI

Mississippi Deaf Service Center
Post Office Box 1698
Jackson, MS 39215
(601) 354-6830 TDD

MISSOURI

Missouri Association of the Deaf
c/o Paraquade, Inc.
5100 Oakland Avenue, #100
St. Louis, MO 63110
(314) 534-0044 TDD

Bridges Beyond Sound
© 1996 Corinne K. Jensema
Paul H. Brookes Publishing Co., Inc.

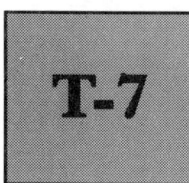

NEBRASKA

Nebraska Association of the Deaf
6231 Read Street
Omaha, NE 68152
(402) 571-7009 V/TDD

NEVADA

Nevada Association of the Deaf
2112 Bavington Drive, #D
Las Vegas, NV 89108
(702) 648-5068 TDD

NEW HAMPSHIRE

NH League for the Hard of Hearing
Post Office Box 6624
Concord, NH 03303
(603) 226-2255 V/TDD

NEW JERSEY

New Jersey Association of the Deaf
1720 Addams Avenue, #L7
Toms River, NJ 08753
(908) 840-6511 TDD

NEW MEXICO

New Mexico Association of the Deaf
Post Office Box 451
Alamogordo, NM 88310
(505) 439-3269 TDD

NEW YORK

Empire State Association of the Deaf
43–74 166th Street
Flushing, NY 11358
(718) 445-0128 TDD

NORTH CAROLINA

North Carolina Association of the Deaf
7801 Corder Avenue
Charlotte, NC 28212
(704) 342-5480 TDD

OHIO

Ohio Association of the Deaf
410 Morrison Road
Columbus, OH 43230
(614) 478-1631 TDD

OKLAHOMA

Tulsa Association of the Deaf
Post Office Box 27523
Tulsa, OK 74149
(918) 582-9584 TDD

OREGON

Deaf Services, Inc.
1020 2nd Avenue, NE, #160
Portland, OR 97232
(503) 232-1025 V/TDD

PENNSYLVANIA

Reading Advancement of the Deaf
538 Franklin Street
Reading, PA 19601
(215) 373-0291 TDD

RHODE ISLAND

Rhode Island Association of the Deaf
37 Lane 2 Laspee Point
Warwick, RI 02888
(401) 463-6915 TDD

Bridges Beyond Sound
© 1996 Corinne K. Jensema
Paul H. Brookes Publishing Co., Inc.

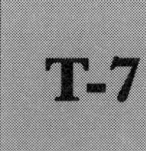

SOUTH CAROLINA

South Carolina Association of the Deaf
1735 Augusta Road
West Columbia, SC 05676
(803) 794-7059 TDD

SOUTH DAKOTA

South Dakota Association of the Deaf
1517 South Wayland
Sioux Falls, SD 57105
(605) 335-7231 V/TDD

TENNESSEE

Hearing Service of Memphis
6133 Poplar Pike
Memphis, TN 38119
(901) 763-4327 V/TDD

TEXAS

Texas Association of the Deaf
Post Office Box 141876
Austin, TX 78714
(512) 280-6517 TDD

UTAH

Community Center for the Deaf
5709 South 1500 Street
West Taylorsville, UT 84123
(801) 288-2159 TDD

VERMONT

Vermont Association of the Deaf
c/o Vermont Rehabilitation Services
103 South Main Street
Waterbury, VT 05676
(802) 241-2199 TDD

VIRGINIA

Virginia Association of the Deaf
7004 Kenfig Drive
Falls Church, VA 22042
(202) 205-7191 TDD

WASHINGTON

Washington Association of the Deaf
Post Office Box 406
Suquamish, WA 98392
(206) 764-3679 V/TDD

WEST VIRGINIA

West Virginia Association of the Deaf
215 East 10th Avenue
Ransom, WV 25438
(304) 725-7466 TDD

WISCONSIN

Wisconsin Association of the Deaf
10890 West Donna Drive
Milwaukee, WI 53224
(414) 355-7498 TDD

Bridges Beyond Sound
© 1996 Corinne K. Jensema
Paul H. Brookes Publishing Co., Inc.

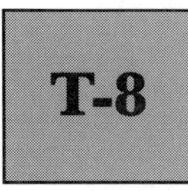

NATIONAL AND INTERNATIONAL ORGANIZATIONS OF AND FOR THE DEAF

The following organizations are sources for more information on all aspects of deafness and hearing loss. The majority have publications that are distributed free of charge or for a small fee to consumers, schools, and teachers. These organizations also can be a resource for speakers, research reports, and deaf awareness activities. Telephones that are accessible by both voice and TDD are indicated by the letters V/TDD beside the number.

ALEXANDER GRAHAM BELL ASSOCIATION FOR THE DEAF, INC. (A.G. BELL)

3417 Volta Place, NW
Washington, DC 20007-2778
(202) 337-5220 V/TDD

A.G. Bell is a consumer organization that espouses oral communication for people with hearing impairments. A.G. Bell publishes a journal, *Volta Review,* an annual monograph, and a newsletter. It also publishes a variety of books and audiovisual materials about the psychological, social, and educational implications of hearing loss. Printed materials are disseminated and inquiries are answered from people with hearing impairments, their families, professionals, and the general public.

AMERICAN ACADEMY OF OTOLARYNGOLOGY—HEAD AND NECK SURGERY (AAO-HNS)

One Prince Street
Alexandria, VA 22314
(703) 836-4444 Voice
(703) 519-1585 TDD

AAO-HNS promotes the art and science of medicine related to otolaryngology (i.e., head and neck surgery), including providing continuing medical education courses and publications. It publishes a variety of pamphlets related to problems with the ear and makes referrals for people with problems to physicians.

AMERICAN ATHLETIC ASSOCIATION OF THE DEAF (AAAD)

3607 Washington Boulevard, #4
Ogden, UT 84403
(801) 393-8710 Voice
(801) 393-7916 TDD

AAAD promotes athletic tournaments in the United States for people who are deaf and coordinates America's involvement in international competitions. The *AAAD Bulletin* is published quarterly.

AMERICAN DEAFNESS AND REHABILITATION ASSOCIATION (ADARA)

Post Office Box 251554
Little Rock, AR 72225
(501) 868-8850 TDD

Bridges Beyond Sound
© 1996 Corinne K. Jensema
Paul H. Brookes Publishing Co., Inc.

ADARA provides referral services regarding careers, university programs, job opportunities, and general information to people with hearing impairments. The national office provides this service free of charge to inquirers. Information regarding legislation, conferences, and workshops can also be obtained through the national office. ADARA publishes the *Journal of the American Deafness and Rehabilitation Association,* a quarterly newsletter entitled *The ADARA Update,* and occasional special publications and monographs. A complete listing of all ADARA publications is available upon request from the national office.

AMERICAN HEARING RESEARCH FOUNDATION (AHRF)

55 East Washington Street, Suite 2022
Chicago, IL 60602
(312) 726-9670 Voice

AHRF is a nonprofit organization that promotes, conducts, and supports medical research into and education about the cause, prevention, and cure of deafness, hearing impairments, and balance disorders. They have a public information and referral system whereby anyone who calls or writes can obtain information on how and where to get medical or educational help. AHRF disseminates brochures on hearing health and research reports for medical specialists on specific hearing problems and balance disorders related to the inner ear.

AMERICAN SOCIETY FOR DEAF CHILDREN (ASDC)

East 10th and Tahlequah
Sulphur, OK 73086
(800) 942-2732 V/TDD

ASDC is a nonprofit, parent-helping-parent organization promoting a positive attitude toward signing and Deaf culture. ASDC provides support, encouragement, and information about deafness to families and supports parents' rights to make choices about communication based on the needs of their children.

AMERICAN SPEECH-LANGUAGE-HEARING ASSOCIATION (ASHA)

10801 Rockville Pike
Rockville, MD 20852
(301) 897-5700 Voice

ASHA provides public information brochures about communication disorders and the roles of speech-language pathologists and audiologists. ASHA has extensive career information in the areas of possible employment, university training programs, and certification requirements. Its publications include: *Journal of Speech and Hearing Research; Journal of Speech and Hearing Disorders; Language, Speech and Hearing Services in Schools; Guide to Professional Services in Speech-Language Pathology and Audiology;* and an *ASHA Directory of Membership.* A monthly magazine, *Asha,* features organizational news, announcements of meetings, job openings, and research reports. Some of the publications are free to members, but any person interested may subscribe or purchase any or all of them. An information and referral service for consumers is accessible via a toll-free helpline (1-800-638-8255).

Bridges Beyond Sound
© 1996 Corinne K. Jensema
Paul H. Brookes Publishing Co., Inc.

T-8

ASSOCIATION OF LATE-DEAFENED ADULTS (ALDA)

10310 Main Street
Post Office Box 274
Fairfax, VA 22030
(815) 899-3049 TDD

ALDA is an organization committed to supporting, educating, representing, and advocating for people who grew up with their hearing and became deaf as adults. ALDA is a membership organization, a self-help support group, and a resource and information center for people who became deaf later in life. Advocacy, self-help, support groups, social activities, outreach, newsletters, consultation, and communication are among the topics of primary focus and concern. They provide a newsletter, *ALDA News,* which is available free of charge to paid members of ALDA.

BETTER HEARING INSTITUTE (BHI)

Post Office Box 1840
Washington, DC 20013
(703) 642-0580 Voice
(800) EAR-WELL V/TDD

BHI is a nonprofit educational organization that implements national public information programs on hearing loss and available medical, surgical, hearing aid, and rehabilitation assistance. It maintains a toll-free "Hearing HelpLine" telephone service that provides information on hearing loss and assistance to callers from anywhere in the United States.

CONFERENCE OF EDUCATIONAL ADMINISTRATORS FOR THE DEAF (CEAD)

800 Florida Avenue, NE
Washington, DC 20002
(202) 651-5015 or (202) 651-5342 V/TDD

CEAD is committed to the improvement of management in programs for the deaf and the maintenance of a continuum of educational options for people who are deaf.

CONVENTION OF AMERICAN INSTRUCTORS OF THE DEAF (CAID)

RIT/NTID
#LBJ2264
Rochester, NY 14623
(716) 475-6201 V/TDD

CAID promotes professional development, communication, and the sharing of information among educators of the deaf. They publish a variety of journals and educational materials.

DEAF ARTISTS OF AMERICA, INC. (DAA)

302 North Goodman Street, #205
Rochester, NY 14607
(716) 244-3460 TDD

Bridges Beyond Sound
© 1996 Corinne K. Jensema
Paul H. Brookes Publishing Co., Inc.

DAA was organized to bring support and recognition to deaf artists. DAA's goals are to collect, publish, and disseminate information about deaf artists; provide cultural and educational opportunities; provide useful services to members; and exhibit and market the works of deaf artists.

DEAFNESS AND COMMUNICATIVE DISORDERS BRANCH (DCDB)

Rehabilitation Services Administration
U.S. Department of Education
600 Independence Avenue, SW, Switzer Building
Washington, DC 20202
(202) 205-8165 V/TDD

DCDB's goal is the promotion of improved and expanded rehabilitation services for people who 1) are deaf, 2) are hard of hearing, 3) are deaf-blind, 4) have speech impairments, or 5) have language disorders. To promote this goal, DCDB engages in a number of activities providing leadership and liaison to national organizations, agencies, and institutions concerned with deafness and communicative disorders; developing policies and standards that improve state rehabilitation agencies' work with clients who have communication impairments; reviewing services provided by state vocational agencies to people who are deaf, hard of hearing, and who have other communication impairments; and providing technical assistance to Rehabilitation Services Administration staff in both central and regional offices.

DEAFNESS RESEARCH FOUNDATION (DRF)

9 East 38th Street, 7th Floor
New York, NY 10016
(212) 684-6559 or (800) 535-3323 V/TDD

The DRF supports and provides grants for research in causes, treatment, and prevention of deafness to hospitals, universities, and nonprofit institutions.

DEAFPRIDE, INC.

1350 Potomac Avenue, SE
Washington, DC 20003
(202) 675-6700 V/TDD

Deafpride, Inc., is a nonprofit organization that works for the human rights of deaf people and their families by bringing together deaf and hearing people and providing opportunities for them to develop their potential as advocates. It offers activities and programs in leadership and advocacy development, family life, bilingual studies and Deaf culture, gaining access to health services, technical assistance, information and referral, and sign language. The organization also provides interpreting services and conducts workshops and in-service training for health services consumers and providers. Deafpride can design programs, conferences, or workshops to meet the specific needs of a group or institution and can provide speakers and panelists from the deaf community. Deafpride has produced a brochure describing its services and a booklet for people who are deaf on how to gain access to medical services.

Bridges Beyond Sound
© 1996 Corinne K. Jensema
Paul H. Brookes Publishing Co., Inc.

THE EAR FOUNDATION

2000 Church Street
Box 111
Nashville, TN 37236
(800) 545-HEAR V/TDD

The Ear Foundation is a national, nonprofit organization committed to leading the effort for better hearing and balance through public and professional educational programs, support services, and applied research.

EPISCOPAL CONFERENCE OF THE DEAF (ECD)

51 Woodale Road
Philadelphia, PA 19118
(215) 247-2245 V/TDD

ECD promotes ministry for people who are deaf through the Episcopal church. It is affiliated with approximately 50 congregations in the United States.

GALLAUDET UNIVERSITY PRESS

800 Florida Avenue, NE
Washington, DC 20002
(800) 451-1073 V/TDD

Gallaudet University Press offers numerous publications about all aspects of deafness. Some recommendations are *Deafness: A Fact Sheet; Resource Listing of Information on Deafness; What Are TDDs?; Guide for TTY—Telephone Communication; Books for Learning Sign Language; Some Signs You Can Learn; A Look at American Sign Language; Directory of National Organizations of and for the Deaf;* and *Locating Sign Language Classes.* Call for a free catalog.

HEARING INFORMATION CENTER

Post Office Box 1880
Media, PA 19063
(800) 622-EARS Voice

The Hearing Information Center provides free information and literature about hearing loss, hearing aids, hearing tests, and rehabilitation. Free local audiological and medical referrals are given to those who request further help. Callers can also be directed to other support groups and organizations for assistance. The center keeps abreast of free hearing tests being offered in different cities and will direct callers when appropriate to the location nearest them.

HEARING LOSS LINK (HLL)

2600 West Peterson Avenue, Suite 202
Chicago, IL 60659
(312) 743-1032 Voice
(312) 743-1007 TDD

Bridges Beyond Sound
© 1996 Corinne K. Jensema
Paul H. Brookes Publishing Co., Inc.

HLL provides counseling, advocacy, referral, and educational services for people who lose their hearing as adults.

INSTITUTE FOR DISABILITIES RESEARCH AND TRAINING, INC. (IDRT)

1299 Lamberton Drive, Suite 200
Silver Spring, MD 20902
(301) 593-2690 V/TDD

IDRT is a corporation that provides training, technical assistance, research and development, advocacy, workshops, and meeting and conference planning services to agencies, organizations, and individuals serving people who are deaf and deaf-blind. IDRT offers training programs on such topics as orientation to deafness, TDD usage, emergency medical treatment for people who have hearing impairments, health care services, how to comply with the ADA, victim services for people with hearing impairments, and 911 response to TDD calls. IDRT can design training programs, conferences, or workshops to meet the specific needs of a group or institution.

INTERNATIONAL CATHOLIC DEAF ASSOCIATION (ICDA)

1707 Richmond Drive
Louisville, KY 40205
(502) 451-4708 TDD

ICDA promotes ministry for people who are Catholic and deaf and responds to spiritually related requests for information worldwide.

INTERNATIONAL LUTHERAN DEAF ASSOCIATION (ILDA)

1333 South Kirkwood Road
St. Louis, MO 63122
(314) 965-9917 V/TDD

ILDA promotes ministry for people who are deaf throughout the Lutheran Church–Missouri Synod.

NATIONAL ASSOCIATION OF THE DEAF (NAD)

814 Thayer Avenue
Silver Spring, MD 20910
(301) 587-1788 Voice
(301) 587-1789 TDD

NAD is a consumer-oriented organization for professionals and laypersons. It recommends and promotes legislation on behalf of deaf people in areas of education, rehabilitation, legal rights for the provision of interpreters, and captioned television. NAD has information on programs and services for the deaf as well as on legislation and legal rights of the deaf. NAD offers a series of workshops on such topics as legal concerns of the deaf, orientation to deafness, leadership training for people who are deaf, and the need for and implementation of mental health services for the deaf. NAD offers a variety of books, audiovisual materials, and merchandise related to deafness and sign language.

Bridges Beyond Sound
© 1996 Corinne K. Jensema
Paul H. Brookes Publishing Co., Inc.

T-8

NATIONAL BLACK DEAF ADVOCATES (NBDA)

1415 Gardenwood Drive
College Park, GA 30349
(404) 997-1489 TDD

NBDA promotes equality, excellence, and empowerment for African American people who are deaf.

NATIONAL CONGRESS OF JEWISH DEAF (NCJD)

33 South Landing Road
Rochester, NY 14610
(716) 387-0762 V/TDD

NCJD advocates for religious, educational, and cultural ideals and fellowship for deaf people who are Jewish.

NATIONAL CUED SPEECH ASSOCIATION (NCSA)

Post Office Box 31345
Raleigh, NC 27622
(919) 828-1218 V/TDD

NCSA is a membership organization that provides advocacy and support regarding the use of cued speech. Information and services are provided for people with hearing impairments, their families and friends, and professionals who work with them.

NATIONAL FRATERNAL SOCIETY OF THE DEAF

1300 West Northwest Highway
Mt. Prospect, IL 60056
(708) 392-9282 Voice
(800) 676-6373 TDD

The society works in the area of insurance and advocacy for people who are deaf.

NATIONAL INFORMATION CENTER ON DEAFNESS (NICD)

Gallaudet University
800 Florida Avenue, NE
Washington, DC 20002
(202) 651-5000 Voice
(202) 651-5052 TDD

NICD is a centralized source of accurate, up-to-date, objective information on topics concerning deafness and hearing loss. NICD responds to questions from the general public and people who have hearing impairments, their families and friends, and professionals who work with them, as well as the general public. NICD collects, develops, and disseminates information on all aspects of hearing loss, as well as the programs and services offered to people who

Bridges Beyond Sound
© 1996 Corinne K. Jensema
Paul H. Brookes Publishing Co., Inc.

are deaf and hard of hearing. NICD provides direct information and printed materials, as well as referrals to other helpful resources when necessary. NICD has developed numerous fact sheets and resource listings on many different topics, such as deafness, TDDs, alerting and communication devices, hearing-ear dogs, financial aid for students with hearing impairments, and reading lists on topics in education of children who are deaf. There is a nominal charge for these publications.

NATIONAL INSTITUTE ON DEAFNESS AND OTHER COMMUNICATION DISORDERS INFORMATION CLEARINGHOUSE

One Communication Avenue
Bethesda, MD 20892-3456
(800) 241-1044 Voice
(800) 241-1055 TDD

The National Institute on Deafness and Other Communication Disorders Information Clearinghouse provides responses to information requests from health professionals, people with hearing impairments, industry, and the public on diseases and disorders of hearing, balance, smell, taste, voice, speech, and language.

NATIONAL TECHNICAL INSTITUTE FOR THE DEAF (NTID)

Rochester Institute of Technology
1 Lomb Memorial Drive
Post Office Box 9887
Rochester, NY 14623
(716) 475-2181 TDD

NTID's Division of Public Affairs provides curriculum materials, communication packages for speech-language pathologists, orientation manuals and information on hearing aids for audiologists and consumers, special bibliographies and other data requested by researchers, and the NTID catalog. The National Center on Employment of the Deaf at NTID offers information and training to employers interested in hiring qualified employees who are deaf.

REGISTRY OF INTERPRETERS FOR THE DEAF, INC. (RID)

8630 Fenton Street, Suite 324
Silver Spring, MD 20910
(301) 608-0050 Voice
(301) 608-0562 TDD

RID publishes and distributes a bimonthly newsletter, *Views,* that focuses on topics of professional concern to interpreters and their clients, as well as publications dealing with the interpreting process. Individuals and organizations may request information about careers in interpreting, the RID National Testing System, finding and hiring an interpreter, tips on using interpreter services, interpreter preparation programs, and interpreter services provider agencies.

Bridges Beyond Sound
© 1996 Corinne K. Jensema
Paul H. Brookes Publishing Co., Inc.

SELF HELP FOR HARD OF HEARING PEOPLE, INC. (SHHH)

7910 Woodmont Avenue, Suite 1200
Bethesda, MD 20814
(301) 657-2248 Voice
(301) 657-2249 TDD

SHHH's goal is to educate people with hearing impairments about hearing loss detection, management, and prevention of further loss, and to develop public and professional acceptance of the needs of people who are hard of hearing. SHHH publishes a bimonthly journal about hearing loss and relevant aids, communication techniques, and programs. Publications are available on a variety of topics. There is a charge for most publications.

TELECOMMUNICATIONS FOR THE DEAF, INC. (TDI)

8719 Colesville Road, Suite 300
Silver Spring, MD 20910
(301) 589-3786 Voice
(301) 589-3006 TDD

TDI serves people with hearing impairments and the general public by assisting them with their telecommunication needs, providing information about telecommunications and deafness, ensuring that everyone has equal access to telecommunications technologies and services, supporting legislation affecting TDD users, and monitoring telecommunications issues and concerns across the United States. TDI publishes an annual international directory of TDD telephone numbers.

TRIPOD GRAPEVINE

2901 North Keystone Street
Burbank, CA 91504
(800) 352-8888 V/TDD Nationwide
(818) 972-2080 California only

TRIPOD provides a national toll-free hotline for parents and people wanting information about raising and educating children who are deaf. It also operates a parent/infant/toddler program, a Montessori preschool, and an inclusive elementary education program for children with hearing impairments.

WORLD FEDERATION OF THE DEAF (WFD)

Illkantie 4
Post Office Box 65
Helsinki- Finland SF004
+358-0-5803-770 TDD

WFD maintains cooperation among national federations of people who are deaf and promotes the exchange of research findings, ideas, and reports. WFD keeps a list of scientists and

Bridges Beyond Sound
© 1996 Corinne K. Jensema
Paul H. Brookes Publishing Co., Inc.

T-8

researchers and publicizes their findings after approval. It also encourages national federations to establish aid programs for people who are deaf in developing countries.

Bridges Beyond Sound
© 1996 Corinne K. Jensema
Paul H. Brookes Publishing Co., Inc.

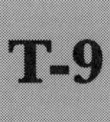

TIPS FOR INCLUDING STUDENTS WHO HAVE HEARING IMPAIRMENTS IN GENERAL CLASSROOMS

Children who have hearing impairments offer many challenges to the general education classroom teacher. The following strategies have been found to be effective by teachers and service personnel who work with these children.

FOR ADMINISTRATORS

- Make sure that your school has a policy that promotes inclusion of students with hearing impairments.
- Make sure that your school enforces inclusion.
- Develop handouts for parents and other community personnel describing your school's efforts to ensure inclusion and the benefits to all students.
- Provide opportunities for all staff to attend in-service training and other growth activities that support information about inclusion and skill building.

FOR TEACHERS

- Be flexible in accepting and creating instructional accommodations.
- Have another student take notes for the child who has a hearing loss or provide copies of your own notes. It is very difficult for a child who is deaf to watch the interpreter, the teacher, and the instructional visual materials, and to take notes at the same time.
- Provide for extra time when giving tests if instructions are given in sign language.
- Write instructions and important information on the chalkboard or on paper for the child.
- Use many visual instructional materials.
- Demonstrate instructions whenever possible.
- Allow for preferential seating.
- Always face the class when speaking. Do not face the chalkboard and verbally give information.
- Do not stand in front of a light source when addressing the child. Lighting should be *on* your face, not casting your face in the shadows and making the child stare into the light.
- Simplify the language you are using if the child does not understand what you are saying.
- Allow and encourage the use of an interpreter (sign or oral). The following should be done if you are using an interpreter:

   Stand near the interpreter when speaking.
   Look directly at the child when speaking to him or her.
   Address all communication to the child when appropriate. Do not say to the interpreter, "Tell him or her...."
   Allow time during question and answer periods or class discussions for the deaf child to take a turn. Remember, the interpreter will always be at least a few words (if not sentences) behind you.

Bridges Beyond Sound
© 1996 Corinne K. Jensema
Paul H. Brookes Publishing Co., Inc.

T-9

Make sure an interpreter is available for all assemblies, field trips, and so forth—not just for classroom work.
Review complex vocabulary and/or concepts with the interpreter prior to instruction.

- Allow and encourage the use of a tutor (e.g., another child in the class, the classroom aide, other service personnel).
- Alert the other children in the class to the fact that one or more of the students has a hearing impairment and work together as a group in deciding how best to accomplish inclusion.
- Comment positively on favorable social interactions that occur among students with and without disabilities.
- Demystify assistive technology (e.g., hearing aids, TDDs) by letting all your students try them.

Bridges Beyond Sound
© 1996 Corinne K. Jensema
Paul H. Brookes Publishing Co., Inc.

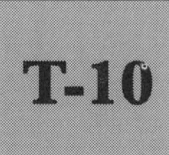

Tips for Evaluating Instructional Materials

As you are aware, children pick up subliminal messages about their teacher's attitude toward people who are ethnically, racially, and religiously different from themselves. It is essential to create role models and positive examples of inclusion for the children to admire. In order to promote inclusion of children with hearing impairments and the acceptance of people without disabilities interacting with all people who have hearing impairments, it is important to make sure that your instructional materials include positive and realistic depictions of people with disabilities. This instructional package has reading suggestions on this topic.

The following are some suggestions for making sure that instructional materials and curricula include accurate depictions of people with hearing impairments:

- Avoid stories that use a paternalistic orientation. Instead, choose stories in which the person's behavior and circumstances are depicted in a normal, competent manner.
- Pick stories in which people with hearing impairments are confronted with situations other than those related to their disability (e.g., divorce, new student at school, getting on a school sports team).
- Select anthologies, book series, and other literature that contain stories with main or support characters who have hearing impairments.
- Avoid materials that treat people who are deaf as a medical anomaly. Deaf people are more than their ears.
- Include Deaf culture as an ethnic minority in your curricula.
- Remember that the personalities of people who have hearing impairments vary just as hearing people's personalities do. Choose materials in which the hearing impairment does not create a "halo effect."
- Make sure that any examples you use include people with hearing impairments.
- Histories should include contributions from people with disabilities. Consider using the "Successful People with Hearing Impairments" handouts included in this instructional package.

Bridges Beyond Sound
© 1996 Corinne K. Jensema
Paul H. Brookes Publishing Co., Inc.

APPLICABLE STUDENT INSTRUCTIONAL MATERIALS

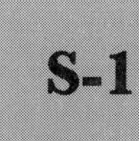

PRETEST

This is a test to see how much you know before you are taught about people who have hearing impairments. Your teacher will test you again when you have finished this instructional unit to see how much you have learned. Follow the instructions for each part of this test.

Circle the letter next to the right answer.

1. People who are deaf _____ .

    a. are all old.

    b. can be any age.

    c. all became deaf before they were born.

    d. all became deaf from listening to rock music too loudly.

2. Children who are deaf _____ .

    a. all go to their neighborhood schools.

    b. all go to schools only for deaf students.

    c. only are in classes for deaf children in their neighborhood schools.

    d. can go to any school where they can get special services.

3. Children who are deaf _____ .

    a. can have parents who are deaf or who can hear.

    b. only have parents who are deaf.

    c. only have parents who can hear.

    d. do not have parents.

4. All children who are deaf _____ .

    a. can speechread well.

    b. know sign language.

    c. wear hearing aids.

    d. need special help to communicate with hearing people.

Bridges Beyond Sound
© 1996 Corinne K. Jensema
Paul H. Brookes Publishing Co., Inc.

S-1

5. _____ is a famous person who is deaf.

   a. Mr. Rogers

   b. Linda Bove

   c. Michael Jordan

   d. Michael Jackson

6. The machine that helps people who are deaf use the telephone is called a _____.

   a. VCR.

   b. TV.

   c. TDD.

   d. Ph.D.

7. The part of a hearing aid that you put in your ear is called _____.

   a. an antenna.

   b. a cord.

   c. a listener.

   d. an ear mold.

8. The sign language used in the United States is called _____.

   a. American Sign Language.

   b. USA Sign Language.

   c. English Sign Language.

   d. Hand Sign Language.

9. The chart used when measuring hearing is called _____.

   a. an audiogram.

   b. a sound level chart.

   c. a hearing status indicator.

   d. a hearing loss graph.

Bridges Beyond Sound
© 1996 Corinne K. Jensema
Paul H. Brookes Publishing Co., Inc.

S-1

10. The outer part of your ear is called the _____ .

   a. earring holder.
   b. eardrum.
   c. cochlea.
   d. pinna.

Decide whether each sentence is true or false. Circle the correct response.

1. People who are deaf can drive. True False
2. People who are deaf always have deaf children. True False
3. People who are deaf always marry other people who are deaf. True False
4. People who are deaf can become teachers. True False
5. People can lose their hearing from accidents. True False
6. Hearing aids can help all people who are deaf. True False
7. A former Miss America is deaf. True False
8. It is easy to speechread. True False
9. The sign language we use in the United States came from France. True False
10. The first deaf teacher of the deaf in the United States was Deaf Smith. True False

Write your answers after each question.

1. If a student in your class was deaf and the interpreter did not show up for class one day, how could you help that student communicate in class?

Bridges Beyond Sound
© 1996 Corinne K. Jensema
Paul H. Brookes Publishing Co., Inc.

S-1

2. If your class is having a party and everyone is to bring something, how could you tell a classmate who is deaf what to bring and what everyone else is bringing?

Bridges Beyond Sound
© 1996 Corinne K. Jensema
Paul H. Brookes Publishing Co., Inc.

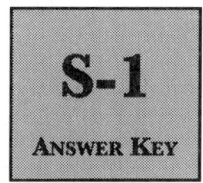

ANSWER KEY

PRETEST

The following are the answers to the Pretest and Posttest.

1. People who are deaf
   b. can be any age.

2. Children who are deaf
   d. can go to any school where they can get special services.

3. Children who are deaf
   a. can have parents who are deaf or who can hear.

4. All children who are deaf
   d. need special help to communicate with hearing people.

5. _____ is a famous person who is deaf.
   b. Linda Bove

6. The machine that helps people who are deaf use the telephone is called a
   c. TDD.

7. The part of a hearing aid that you put in your ear is called
   d. an ear mold.

8. The sign language used in the United States is called
   a. American Sign Language.

9. The chart used when measuring hearing is called
   a. an audiogram.

10. The outer part of your ear is called the
    d. pinna.

Decide whether each sentence is true or false. Circle the correct response.

1. People who are deaf can drive.   (True)   False

2. People who are deaf always have deaf children.   True   (False)

3. People who are deaf always marry other people who are deaf.   True   (False)

Bridges Beyond Sound
© 1996 Corinne K. Jensema
Paul H. Brookes Publishing Co., Inc.

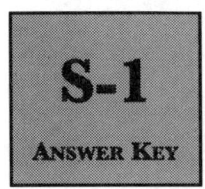

S-1
ANSWER KEY

4. People who are deaf can become teachers. (True) False

5. People can lose their hearing from accidents. (True) False

6. Hearing aids can help all people who are deaf. True (False)

7. A former Miss America is deaf. (True) False

8. It is easy to speechread. True (False)

9. The sign language we use in the United States came from France. (True) False

10. The first deaf teacher of the deaf in the United States was Deaf Smith. True (False)

Write your answers after each question.

1. If a student in your class was deaf and the interpreter did not show up for class one day, how could you help that student communicate in class?

    Look for answers such as:

    a. Take notes for the student.

    b. Hire a freelance interpreter.

    c. Demonstrate instructions to the student.

    d. Use more visual instructional materials.

    e. Have the teacher give his or her notes to the student.

2. If your class is having a party and everyone is to bring something, how could you tell a classmate who is deaf what to bring and what everyone else is bringing?

    Look for answers such as:

    a. Write down each child's name and what he or she is bringing.

    b. If the student cannot read, point to each child and draw pictures of what each child is bringing.

    c. Point to each child and then to samples of what each child is to bring.

    d. Point to each child and act out what each is to bring.

Bridges Beyond Sound
© 1996 Corinne K. Jensema
Paul H. Brookes Publishing Co., Inc.

S-2

FACTS AND MYTHS ABOUT DEAFNESS

Circle "yes" or "no" for each statement.

1. Can people who are deaf drive?	Yes No
2. Do all people who are deaf use sign language?	Yes No
3. Can people who are deaf see better than hearing people?	Yes No
4. Can people who are deaf get married?	Yes No
5. Can people who are deaf marry hearing people?	Yes No
6. Can people who are deaf go to movies and watch TV?	Yes No
7. Can people who are deaf go to college?	Yes No
8. Do all people who are deaf wear hearing aids?	Yes No
9. Can people who are deaf ride bikes?	Yes No
10. Can all people who are deaf speechread well?	Yes No
11. Can people who are deaf listen to music and dance?	Yes No
12. Do parents who are deaf always have children who are deaf?	Yes No
13. Can people who are deaf be teachers?	Yes No
14. Do people who are deaf need to read braille?	Yes No
15. Are there any famous people who are deaf?	Yes No
16. Do you know anyone with a hearing problem?	Yes No
17. Can anyone lose his or her hearing?	Yes No

Bridges Beyond Sound
© 1996 Corinne K. Jensema
Paul H. Brookes Publishing Co., Inc.

S-2

18. Are there any students with hearing impairments at your school?   Yes   No

19. Do children who are deaf grow up to be hearing adults?   Yes   No

20. Can people who are deaf read and write?   Yes   No

21. Can people who are deaf have children?   Yes   No

22. Do children who are deaf play games?   Yes   No

23. Can people who are deaf talk?   Yes   No

24. Can people who are deaf work?   Yes   No

25. Can people who are deaf use the telephone?   Yes   No

Bridges Beyond Sound
© 1996 Corinne K. Jensema
Paul H. Brookes Publishing Co., Inc.

S-2 ANSWER KEY

FACTS AND MYTHS ABOUT DEAFNESS

Most of the answers for this exercise can be found by reading the "Fact Sheet About Hearing Loss and People Who Have Hearing Impairments" (T-1) and "Questions Commonly Asked by Children About People Who Have Hearing Impairments" (T-2). The correct answers are listed below. You may want to use this exercise to initiate a discussion about each topic and how people with hearing impairments may need extra assistance or adaptive devices to do certain activities, but that this does not indicate that they are less intelligent or less capable. For those questions that have "no" answers, discuss with the class why the answer is no.

Circle "yes" or "no" for each statement.

1. Can people who are deaf drive? — **Yes** / No
2. Do all people who are deaf use sign language? — Yes / **No**
3. Can people who are deaf see better than hearing people? — Yes / **No**
4. Can people who are deaf get married? — **Yes** / No
5. Can people who are deaf marry hearing people? — **Yes** / No
6. Can people who are deaf go to movies and watch TV? — **Yes** / No
7. Can people who are deaf go to college? — **Yes** / No
8. Do all people who are deaf wear hearing aids? — Yes / **No**
9. Can people who are deaf ride bikes? — **Yes** / No
10. Can all people who are deaf speechread well? — Yes / **No**
11. Can people who are deaf listen to music and dance? — **Yes** / No
12. Do parents who are deaf always have children who are deaf? — Yes / **No**
13. Can people who are deaf be teachers? — **Yes** / No
14. Do people who are deaf need to read braille? — Yes / **No**

Bridges Beyond Sound
© 1996 Corinne K. Jensema
Paul H. Brookes Publishing Co., Inc.

S-2 ANSWER KEY

15. Are there any famous people who are deaf? (Yes) No

16. Do you know anyone with a hearing problem? Yes No

17. Can anyone lose his or her hearing? (Yes) No

18. Are there any students with hearing impairments at your school? Yes No

19. Do children who are deaf grow up to be hearing adults? Yes (No)

20. Can people who are deaf read and write? (Yes) No

21. Can people who are deaf have children? (Yes) No

22. Do children who are deaf play games? (Yes) No

23. Can people who are deaf talk? (Yes) No

24. Can people who are deaf work? (Yes) No

25. Can people who are deaf use the telephone? (Yes) No

Bridges Beyond Sound
© 1996 Corinne K. Jensema
Paul H. Brookes Publishing Co., Inc.

S-3

A World without Sound

Follow the directions below:

1. Write down all the sounds you hear around you right now and the sounds you enjoy listening to.

Sounds heard	Sounds enjoyed

2. Look at the list. Cross out all of the sounds you think you could live without or that are not necessary in your life.

3. Share your list with the rest of the class and explain why you crossed out what you did.

Bridges Beyond Sound
© 1996 Corinne K. Jensema
Paul H. Brookes Publishing Co., Inc.

S-3

4. Write down ways you could compensate for not hearing the following sounds:
   - Sirens: _____
   - Your parents calling you to dinner: _____
   - Instructions from your teacher: _____
   - Your friend calling you on the telephone: _____
   - Cars: _____
   - A smoke detector: _____
   - The doorbell: _____
   - The television: _____

5. Pick a partner and act out the following roles:
   - Partner 1 is a child who is deaf. Partner 2 is a hearing friend.
     Partner 2 (the hearing friend) must give Partner 1 a warning about a danger. Partner 2 can pick the danger he or she wants to use. Some ideas include a car coming, a fire in the house, or the tub overflowing in a bathroom.
   - Partner 1 is a child who is deaf. Partner 2 is a hearing teacher.
     Partner 2 (the hearing teacher) must tell Partner 1 what the homework assignment is. Partner 2 can make up his or her own homework assignment.
   - Partner 1 is a child who is deaf. Partner 2 is a hearing friend.
     Partner 2 (the hearing friend) must tell Partner 1 about a field trip. Partner 2 can pick his or her own trip destination.

Bridges Beyond Sound
© 1996 Corinne K. Jensema
Paul H. Brookes Publishing Co., Inc.

S-4

FACT SHEET ABOUT HEARING LOSS AND PEOPLE WHO HAVE HEARING IMPAIRMENTS

The following are three vocabulary words that you should know when talking about people who have a hearing loss:

- **Deafness**   A condition that makes a person unable to hear well enough for everyday activities
- **Deaf**   Having a hearing impairment that is so great that a person cannot understand speech even while wearing a hearing aid
- **Hard of hearing**   Having a hearing impairment that makes it difficult, but not impossible, to understand speech

There are many factors concerning a hearing loss that affect a person's behavior or ability to do things. Defining a hearing loss is very difficult because so many factors are involved. All of these factors make each person who has a hearing impairment unique. These factors include the following:

- When the person became deaf
- How great the hearing loss is
- The type of hearing loss
- The condition of the loss (e.g., Is it temporary, permanent, or changing?)
- The personality of the person
- The person's surroundings
- The person's family

All ethnic groups have terms that they like and dislike. For example, many African American people do not want to be called *Black*; they want to be called *African American*. People with hearing losses have the same kind of feelings. Sometimes people do not want to be called *deaf* because it reminds them of the phrase "deaf and dumb." Other people take great pride in the term *deaf* and want to be known as a member of Deaf culture. Some of these people take offense if they are called *hearing impaired*. People with any type of hearing loss, mild to profound, should be referred to as having a hearing impairment or loss.

DID YOU KNOW THAT...

Approximately 24 million Americans have a hearing loss. A hearing loss can range from mild to profound and makes each individual special. Hearing impairments affect people of all ages and can develop at any point in their lives. Some people are born with a hearing loss. These people have a **congenital** loss. Others

Bridges Beyond Sound
© 1996 Corinne K. Jensema
Paul H. Brookes Publishing Co., Inc.

S-4

lose their hearing as the result of an illness or injury. Most **acquired** hearing losses are caused by getting old. A lot of older people have a hearing loss.

IDENTIFYING A HEARING LOSS

Hearing loss is defined by the **degree** of loss and the **type** of loss. These two factors are decided through audiological testing, which is testing of the ear. The person who does the testing is usually an **audiologist.** Testing is done using earphones placed over a person's ears. The audiologist sends **tones** (sounds) through the earphones to one ear at a time. These tones are different **frequencies** (high or low) and **intensities** (loud or soft). Frequency is measured in **Hertz** (Hz), and intensity is measured in **Decibels** (dB). The quietest sound the person can hear at each frequency is marked on a graph called an **audiogram.** Tones are normally presented at 250, 500, 1,000, 2,000, 4,000, and sometimes 8,000 Hz. The normal threshold of hearing (the intensity at which a tone is heard) is between 0 dB and 15 dB. Usually, 0 dB is the quietest a person can hear a tone of 1,000 Hz. If the tone is not heard, the intensity (loudness) is increased until the person either hears the tone or feels the tone (if it is really loud). Marks are made on the audiogram for both ears.

DECIDING WHAT KIND OF HEARING LOSS A PERSON HAS

After audiological testing has been completed, the audiogram is read by the audiologist, who will define both the type of loss and the degree of loss.

The **type** of hearing loss refers to the cause of the loss. The audiogram will indicate which part of the ear is damaged. Some hearing losses can be fixed by surgery or helped by a hearing aid, but not all people can be helped. There are three types of hearing loss: conductive, sensorineural, and mixed.

A **conductive** loss means that the loss is caused by problems in the outer or middle ear. Sometimes, this type of loss can be corrected by surgery. Sometimes people with conductive losses can hear themselves but not other people. Ear infections and fluid in the middle ear can cause a temporary conductive hearing loss.

A **sensorineural** loss means that the hearing loss was caused by problems in the inner ear or auditory nerve. This type of hearing loss cannot be fixed. With this type of loss, a person may not be able to hear his or her own voice or other sounds.

A **mixed** loss means that the hearing loss is conductive and sensorineural. This type of loss is different from person to person.

Bridges Beyond Sound
© 1996 Corinne K. Jensema
Paul H. Brookes Publishing Co., Inc.

S-4

The **degree** (severity) of hearing loss means how loud a sound has to be for a person to hear it. The **hearing threshold** is the quietest sound a person can hear at the frequencies measured by the audiogram. There are six categories of severity of loss: normal, slight, mild, moderate, severe, and profound.

- People who have **normal** hearing have a hearing threshold (loudness level) of 0 dB–15 dB. At this level, an individual can hear all speech sounds.
- People with a **slight** hearing loss have a hearing threshold of 15 dB–25 dB. At this level, an individual can hear all vowel sounds but may not hear some unvoiced consonants, such as *f, t, p, k, ch, h,* and/or *s*. Children with this amount of loss may have some problems learning to speak.
- People with a **mild** hearing loss have a hearing threshold of 25 dB–40 dB. At this level, a person can hear only some vowel sounds and loud voiced consonants, such as *l, m,* and/or *n*. This amount of loss can cause problems learning speech and language, paying attention, and understanding what other people say.
- People with a **moderate** hearing loss have a hearing threshold of 40 dB–65 dB. At this level, a person cannot hear most speech sounds at a normal conversational level. This amount of loss also can cause problems with learning speech and language, paying attention, and understanding what other people say.
- People with a **severe** hearing loss have a hearing threshold of 65 dB–95 dB. At this level, an individual can hear *no* speech sounds without a hearing aid. This kind of hearing loss may cause severe problems with learning language, doing well in school, and paying attention.
- People with a **profound** hearing loss have a hearing threshold of 95 dB or higher. (The threshold of pain is 130 dB; any sound at this level is painful to a person with normal hearing.) At this level, a person hears no speech sounds and few environmental sounds. This kind of loss may cause serious problems with learning language, doing schoolwork, and paying attention.

EFFECTS OF HEARING LOSS

Hearing impairments are not easy to understand. People who have hearing impairments have complicated problems when communicating. The most important thing to remember is that having a hearing loss makes understanding spoken language very difficult. Many people who have hearing impairments cannot hear others speak or hear their own voices.

A hearing loss also affects a person's ability to learn spoken language. A baby with a hearing loss will have more problems learning language than an adult who becomes deaf.

Bridges Beyond Sound
© 1996 Corinne K. Jensema
Paul H. Brookes Publishing Co., Inc.

S-4

The **nature** of a hearing loss means how long it will last and the cause. A hearing loss can be temporary, permanent, fluctuating, or degenerative (it gets worse over time).

- You can get a **temporary** hearing loss at any time. It can last a day or a few years. These hearing losses are caused by blows to the head, being around loud noises, sickness, or ear infections.
- You can be born with a **permanent** hearing loss or get one during your life. This type of loss never goes away. You can inherit a permanent loss or an accident can cause one.
- **Fluctuating** hearing losses change from day to day. You can get them at any time. A person who has a fluctuating hearing loss will not be able to hear the same thing from day to day.
- A **degenerative** hearing loss gets worse over time. Sometimes the change is fast and sometimes it is slow. This type of hearing loss can also be hereditary or caused by an illness or accident.

The **age of onset** refers to when the loss happened. There are three categories describing the age of onset: congenital, acquired/adventitious, and presbycusis.

- A **congenital** hearing loss means a person's hearing loss was present at birth. People who have a congenital loss have the hardest time learning speech and spoken language.
- An **acquired/adventitious** hearing loss can happen or develop at any time during a person's life. Some people lose their hearing as young children, some as teenagers, and many as adults. This type of hearing loss can be caused by heredity, illness, or accident. The extent to which the hearing loss affects the person depends on age, stage of development, and personality. In most cases, younger people have more difficulties than older people.
- **Presbycusis** is the word used to describe a hearing loss that occurs as people grow old. Sometimes it is hard for older people to accept that they have lost their hearing and to wear hearing aids.

The **emotional status** of an individual who has a hearing loss can greatly affect his or her ability to deal with life and be successful. Each person who has a hearing loss deals with the loss and its effect on his or her life. A person with an acquired loss usually has a more difficult time accepting the hearing loss than a person who was born with it. A hearing loss affects all aspects of a person's life. People with acquired hearing loss may have problems communicating with their families, being accepted by others, continuing to do well at work or school, doing

Bridges Beyond Sound
© 1996 Corinne K. Jensema
Paul H. Brookes Publishing Co., Inc.

daily chores without help, learning to wear hearing aids, and enjoying their usual forms of entertainment.

The reason for a hearing loss may cause other disabilities as well. Having more disabilities can make more problems for the person who is deaf. Some people who have hearing impairments may also have mental retardation, vision impairments, learning disabilities, emotional impairments, cerebral palsy, mental illness, or other physical disabilities.

DEAF CULTURE

For centuries, people who are deaf have developed their own *deaf community*. This community has its own history and heritage just like any other ethnic group of people. They have their own language, and they share many of the same experiences throughout their lives. Their heritage is passed down from parents who are deaf to their children and from one person who is deaf to another through deaf humor and signlore.

Deaf Humor

Deaf humor, an important part of Deaf culture, takes a look at the world from the point of view of a person who has a hearing impairment. Deaf people laugh at themselves and the situations they find in everyday life. Many jokes are visual plays on words, like verbal jokes play on words. Deaf jokes are usually hard for people who can hear to understand.

Signlore

Signlore, another important part of Deaf culture, is a way of handing down stories, events, and finger games in sign language. These stories are not written, but passed on manually (on the hands) from one person who is deaf to another. Signlore and humor are known among people who are deaf just as nursery rhymes and jokes are known among people who can hear. Deaf culture is very rich and people who are deaf feel very proud to be a part of the deaf community.

DEAF EDUCATION

Every parent who has a child with a hearing impairment has the same goal for his or her child. Parents want their children to learn to communicate and reach their highest abilities. The educational methods they choose to help their children reach this goal vary.

There are generally two different ways of educating children who are deaf—the **oral (aural) method** and the **manual method.** There is no exact way of deciding which way is best for a child. Each family must decide on its own.

Bridges Beyond Sound
© 1996 Corinne K. Jensema
Paul H. Brookes Publishing Co., Inc.

S-4

Oral Method

The oral (aural) method teaches speechreading and oral speech to children with hearing impairments through the use of hearing aids and training by using the hearing the child has left. If the training is successful, this method is good because the child learns to understand and speak English. Knowing how to speak English helps a child function in the hearing world. A person educated in the oral method often has more educational and job choices.

Another advantage of this method is that family members do not have to learn a new form of communication. With the oral method, the family is taught how to help the child learn language through speechreading and residual hearing training.

One of the big problems with the oral method is that not all children learn oral and aural skills well enough to communicate with people who can hear. Many oral children attend inclusive schools. They may have problems communicating with their teachers and classmates, or they may be the only child with a hearing impairment at school. This makes them feel different from other people. Also, because they did not learn sign language, they will have problems communicating with other people who are deaf.

If the child is unsuccessful, it is hard to change to the manual method. Sometimes oral adults say they do not feel like a part of the hearing world or the deaf world. This can affect their self-confidence.

Manual Method

The manual method teaches sign language to children with hearing impairments. It also encourages the use of hearing aids. The sign language used most commonly in the United States is American Sign Language (ASL). ASL is a true language, with its own grammar and rules of use.

The best advantage of the manual method is that a child can always see the language. It allows a child to learn language at about the same rate as a hearing child. Studies show that deaf children of deaf parents who communicate using sign language do better in school than deaf children who have parents who can hear. This is because they learn language from birth. These children develop a lot like hearing children in hearing families.

The manual method lets a child learn without having communication difficulties. This method also lets a child become part of Deaf culture. Most schools that use ASL will also teach students about Deaf culture.

One problem with the manual method is that ASL is a language different from English. ASL is a visual language. Communication is based on how the eye

Bridges Beyond Sound
© 1996 Corinne K. Jensema
Paul H. Brookes Publishing Co., Inc.

S-4

sees. English is an auditory language. It is based on how the ear hears and the mouth works. Often, people who are taught through the manual method do not read and write English well. This may lead to problems in higher education and in the workplace.

Another problem is that only a small part of the population uses ASL. People who use ASL may have problems communicating with the hearing world and depend on a family member, friend, or sign language interpreter to communicate with hearing people. This may limit a person's independence.

When a hearing family with a child who has a hearing impairment chooses the manual method, the family members must also learn sign language. This may be a problem if the family does not learn sign language as quickly as the child.

Other deaf education methods include **cued speech** and **total communication.** Cued speech was developed by Dr. Orin Cornett at Gallaudet University. This is a visual system. It shows all of the sounds in the English language through hand signals. It is not a language like ASL. It is a system to improve oral communication.

Total communication is a philosophy that says to use any and all communication methods that help a child who has a hearing impairment to communicate. Usually, **simultaneous communication** (speech and a manual English method) is used for conversations.

Bridges Beyond Sound
© 1996 Corinne K. Jensema
Paul H. Brookes Publishing Co., Inc.

S-5

SAMPLE AUDIOGRAM

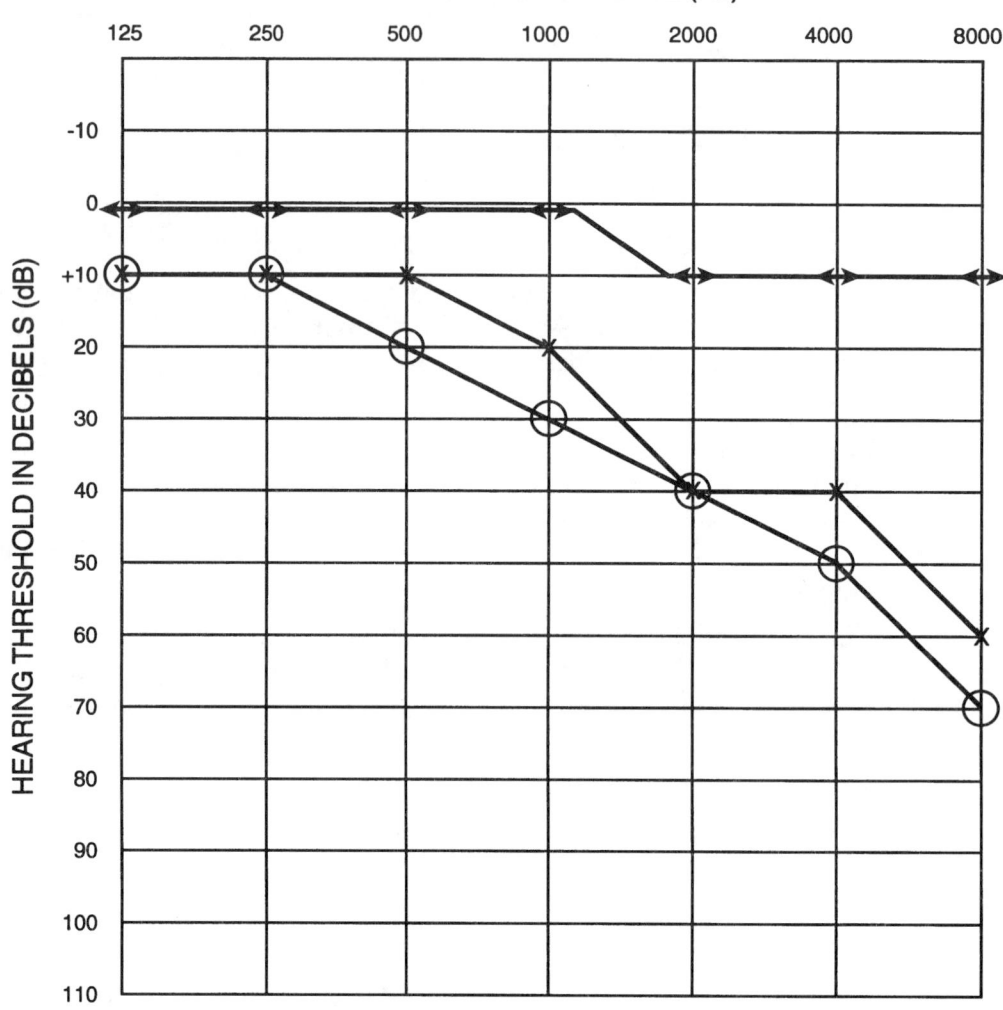

S-6

AUDIOGRAM WITH DEGREES OF HEARING LOSS

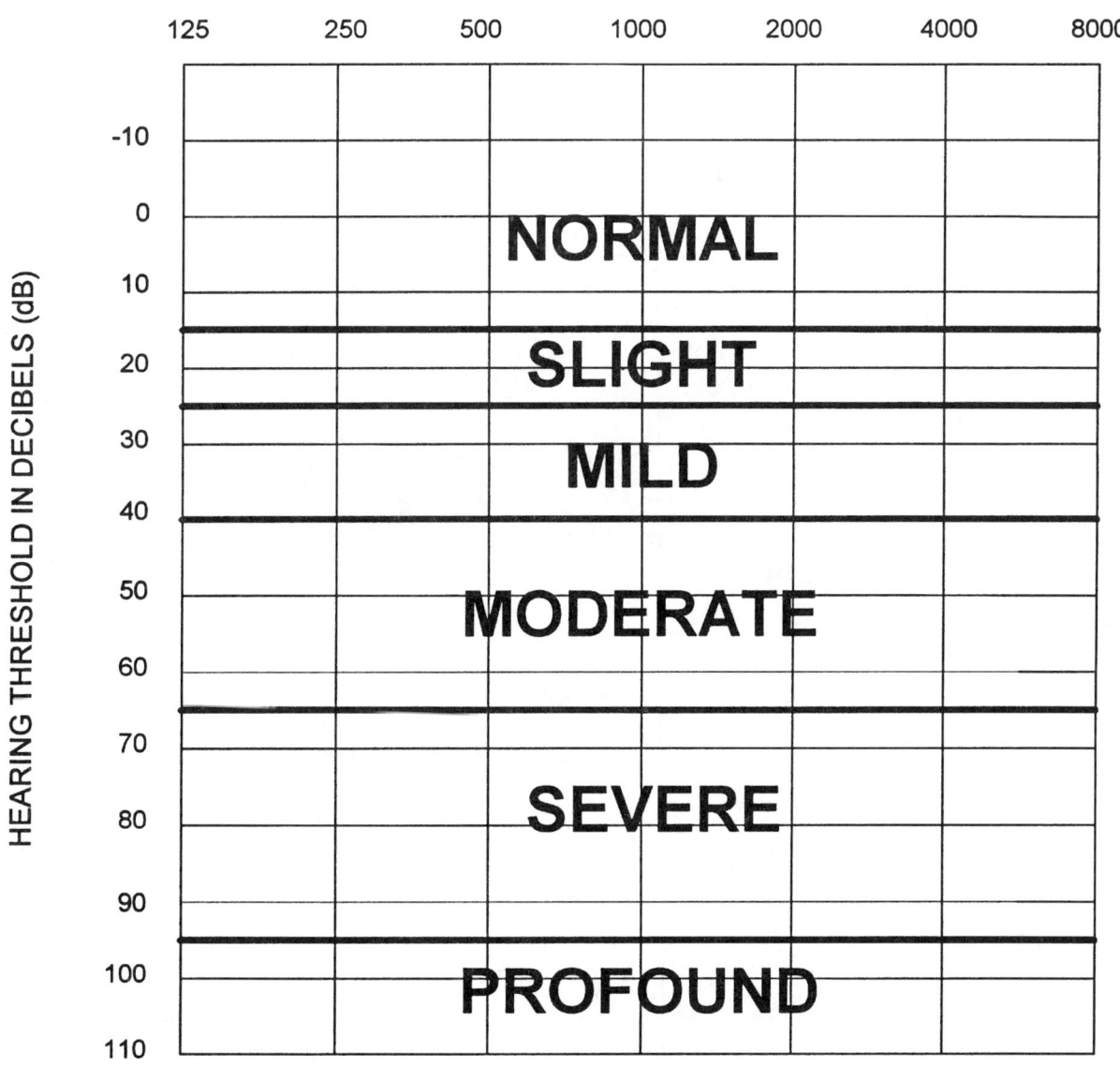

Bridges Beyond Sound
© 1996 Corinne K. Jensema
Paul H. Brookes Publishing Co., Inc.

Audiogram of Environmental and Speech Sounds

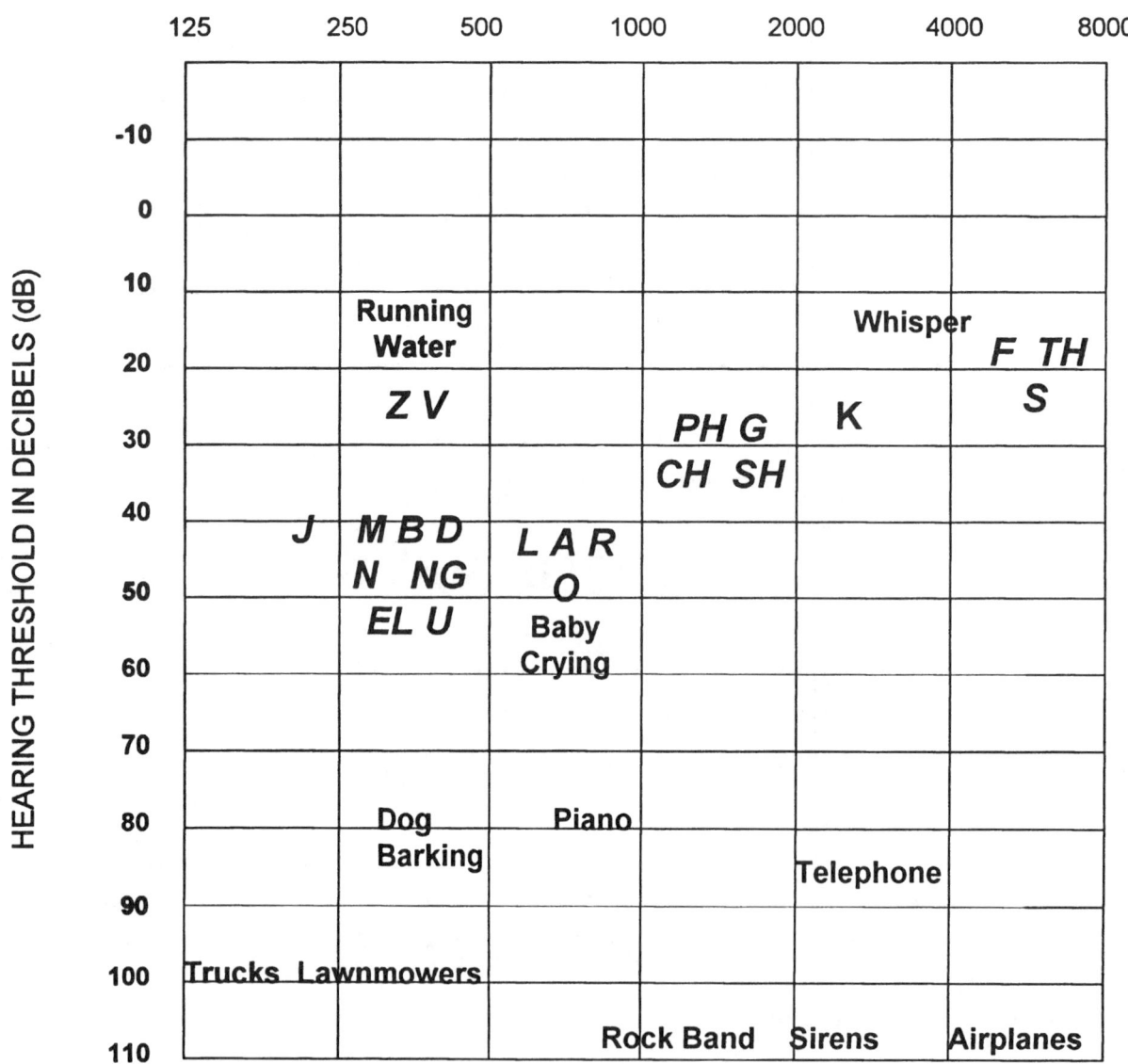

Sounds louder than 90 dB can cause temporary or permanent damage to hearing if you are around them for a long time.

Bridges Beyond Sound
© 1996 Corinne K. Jensema
Paul H. Brookes Publishing Co., Inc.

S-8

How the Ear Works

The ear has many different parts. Together they form the **outer, middle,** and **inner** portions of the ear. The **outer ear** is the part of the ear that you can see. The part on the side of your head is called the **pinna.** The pinna acts like a satellite dish, catching sound waves and directing them into the **ear canal.** The ear canal directs the sound waves to the eardrum. The **eardrum** is a thin membrane that is stretched tight across the end of the ear canal, just like the top part of a drum.

When sound waves hit the eardrum, they make it vibrate. These vibrations move bones that are behind the eardrum in the **middle ear.** The middle ear is a space filled with air. Sometimes liquid fills up the middle ear and people get earaches and ear infections. Some children have to have special tubes put in their ears by doctors to stop the liquid from filling up the middle ear space. The **eustachian tube** is a part of the middle ear. It connects the middle ear to an area in the back of your throat. That is why sometimes when you have a sore throat, you might have an earache, too. The eustachian tube allows air to get into the middle ear, which helps stop fluid from filling up the middle ear. There are three very small bones in the middle ear called the **hammer, anvil,** and **stirrup.** These are the smallest bones in a person's body. The three bones are connected to each other. The eardrum vibrates and moves the hammer. The hammer moves the anvil, and the anvil moves the stirrup.

The stirrup bone is connected to the **round window,** which is the beginning of the **inner ear.** When the stirrup bone moves, it makes the round window vibrate. The round window is part of the **cochlea.** The cochlea is a fluid-filled tube, lined with thousands of hairs, that is curled up like a snail shell. When the round window vibrates, it moves the fluid in the cochlea. The hairs in the cochlea move back and forth when the fluid moves, just like seaweed does in the ocean. Each hair movement sends a signal through the **auditory nerve** to the brain. The hairs are attached to nerves and the nerves join to form the auditory nerve, which goes to the brain. The brain interprets the signal as the kind of sound that was received by the ear.

Bridges Beyond Sound
© 1996 Corinne K. Jensema
Paul H. Brookes Publishing Co., Inc.

S-9

DIAGRAM OF THE EAR

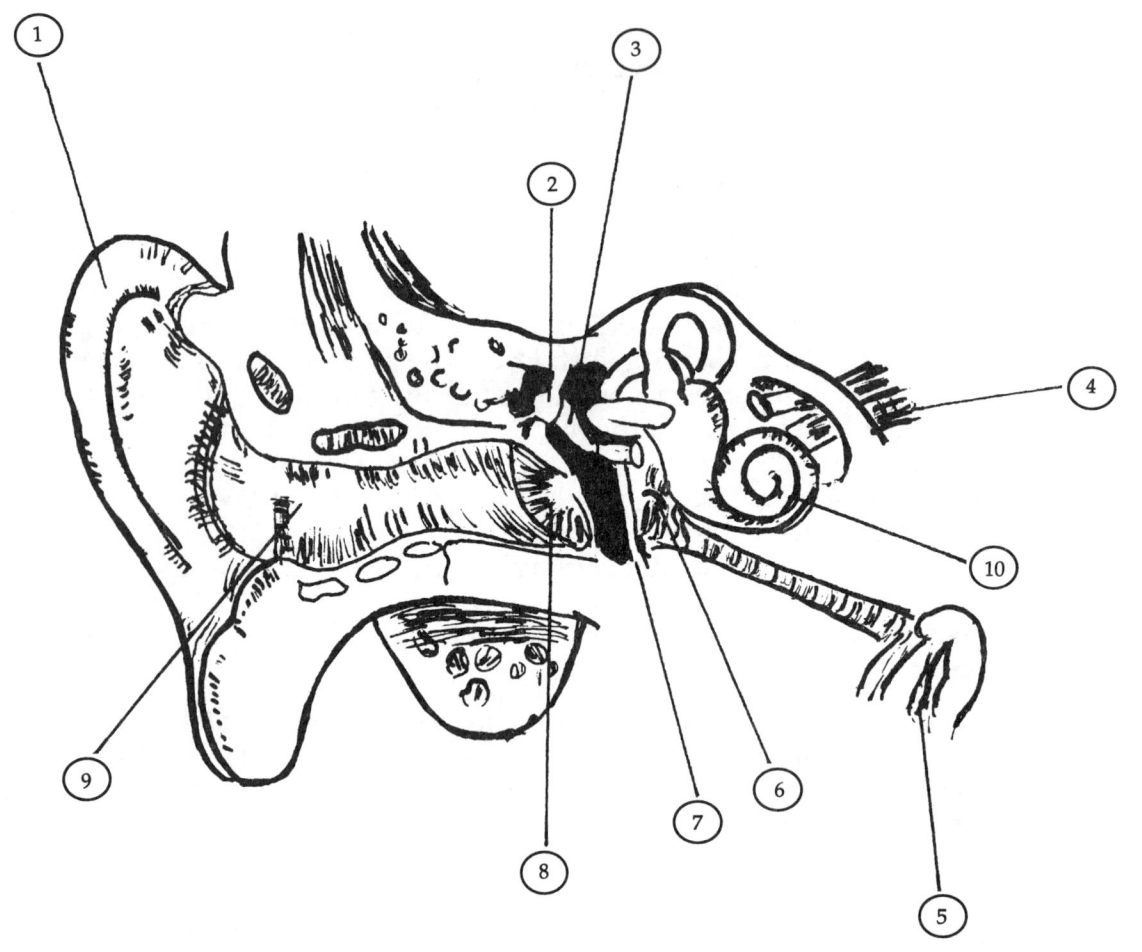

1. _____
2. _____
3. _____
4. _____
5. _____
6. _____
7. _____
8. _____
9. _____
10. _____

Bridges Beyond Sound
© 1996 Corinne K. Jensema
Paul H. Brookes Publishing Co., Inc.

S-9
ANSWER KEY

DIAGRAM OF THE EAR

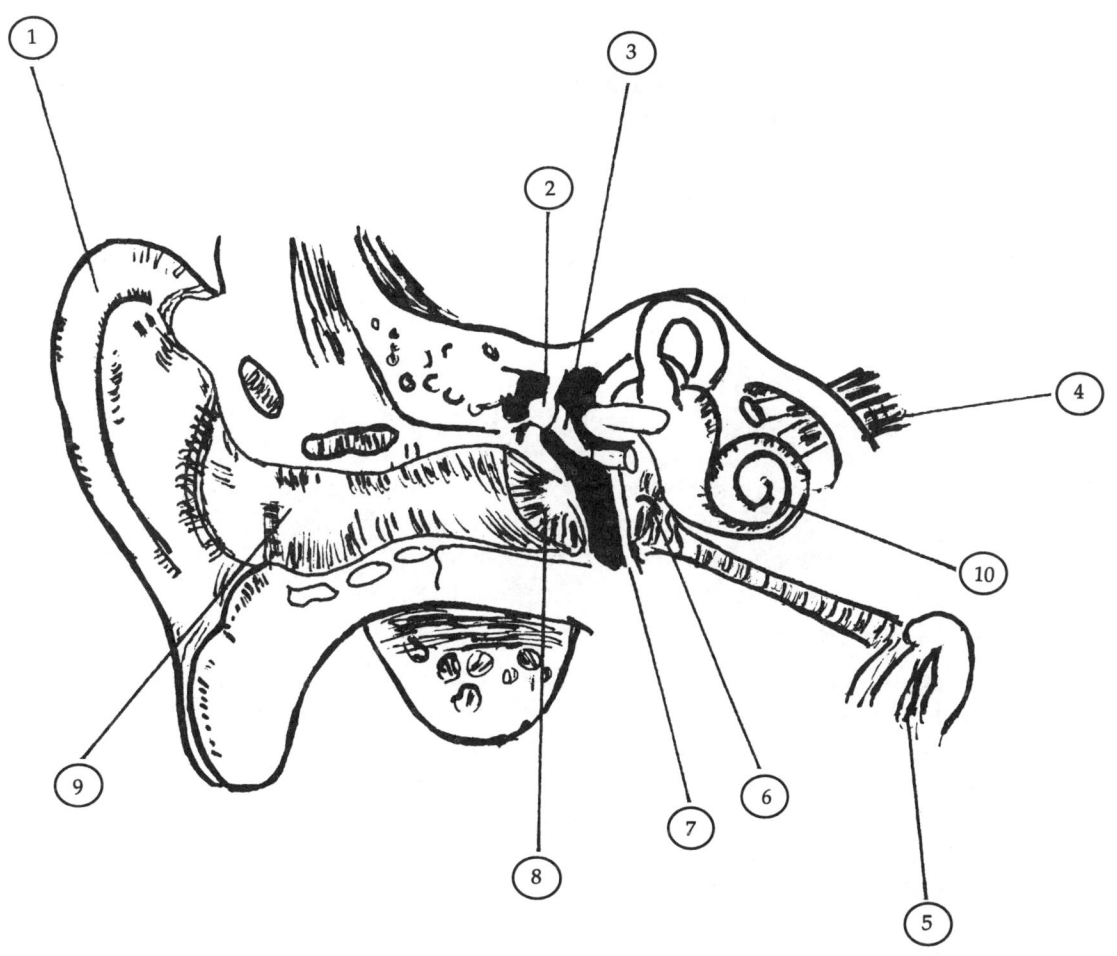

1. pinna

2. hammer

3. anvil

4. auditory nerve

5. eustachian tube

6. round window

7. stirrup

8. eardrum

9. ear canal

10. cochlea

Bridges Beyond Sound
© 1996 Corinne K. Jensema
Paul H. Brookes Publishing Co., Inc.

S-10

Technology Used by People Who Have Hearing Impairments

Many people with hearing impairments cannot use some of the machines that people with normal hearing use to make their lives easier. Some examples are alarm clocks, telephones, doorbells, televisions, fire alarms, and burglar alarms. People who have hearing impairments cannot use many of these devices because they make sounds that they cannot hear. However, there are many helpful devices that people who have hearing impairments use to make up for not being able to hear these sounds.

HEARING AIDS

Hearing aids are electronic machines that make sounds louder. Some people who have a hearing loss use a hearing aid to help them hear important sounds like traffic and fire alarms, but some people cannot use them at all. The hearing loss is too severe for a hearing aid to help. People can wear either one or two hearing aids. Each person's hearing is different, so a hearing aid must be fitted just like eyeglasses. There are three kinds of hearing aids: in-the-ear aids, behind-the-ear aids, and body aids.

In-the-ear aids are very small and fit inside the ear canal. These are mostly used by older people who have lost some of their hearing over the years. **Behind-the-ear aids** are the most common type of hearing aids, although this is changing as in-the-ear aids become more powerful. These fit behind the ear and have a tube that connects to another part that fits inside the ear. A **body aid** looks like a small radio and is worn on a person's chest. A body aid has a wire that is connected to either one or two receivers worn inside the ear.

ALARM CLOCKS

People with hearing impairments need to get up at certain times in the morning just like everyone else, but regular alarm clocks will not wake them. There are alarm clocks that set off a flashing light or vibrate the bed to wake a person. Just like with sound alarms, these do not work for everyone.

TELECOMMUNICATION DEVICES FOR THE DEAF (TDDs)

Telecommunication devices for the deaf (TDDs) are machines that can be hooked up to the telephone and that provide a way for people with hearing impairments to use the telephone. A TDD has a keyboard and a small screen like a computer. People can type messages to each other over the telephone using this device. Because only one person can type on a TDD at a time, there are codes that each writer uses to tell the other person when he or she is finished or wants a

Bridges Beyond Sound
© 1996 Corinne K. Jensema
Paul H. Brookes Publishing Co., Inc.

S-10

response. This system works only when there is a TDD on each end. A person cannot talk to a TDD, and a TDD cannot talk to a person. People with hearing impairments can use TDDs to call almost anywhere. They can even call 911 when there is an emergency to get the rescue squad, police, or fire department.

If a person with a hearing impairment wants to call someone who does not have a TDD, he or she can use the state relay service. This service provides a way for people who have TDDs to communicate with people who do not. A person calls the relay service either on the telephone or on a TDD and gives the number of the person he or she wants to call to the operator at the relay center. The operators are called *communication assistants.* The communication assistant will then call the other person and use both a TDD and his or her voice to communicate a message between the two callers.

ALERTING DEVICES

People who can hear react to the sounds they can hear, such as the telephone or doorbell ringing, someone knocking on the door, a fire or burglar alarm, or a baby crying. People with hearing impairments want to know about these same events, but they may not hear the sounds. Alerting devices have been designed to help them. Alerting devices are usually flashing lights attached to the telephone, doorbell, door, or fire or burglar alarm. Flashing lights will blink on and off to signal what is happening when the telephone or doorbell rings, someone knocks on the door, or an alarm goes off. Different lights flash for different sounds so that the person will know exactly why the lights are flashing and can respond correctly.

There is also a device called a *baby cry detector* that a person can put near a baby's crib (like a baby monitor) that will flash a light when the baby cries. This allows a person with a hearing impairment the same freedom a baby monitor does for a hearing person.

CLOSED-CAPTIONED TELEVISION

Closed captioning is a system in which the words spoken on television are printed at the bottom of the television screen. You must have a special machine called a *decoder* or a television with a built-in decoder to see the printed words on television shows. Not all television shows are closed captioned. The letters CC on the screen at the beginning of a television show indicate that the show is closed captioned.

Before closed captioning was invented, people with hearing impairments could only see what was happening on television. They could not understand what was being said. Many people tried speechreading the people on television,

Bridges Beyond Sound
© 1996 Corinne K. Jensema
Paul H. Brookes Publishing Co., Inc.

S-10

but this was very difficult to do. Sometimes the television show does not show the person who is talking or the person has his or her back to the camera. Try watching television with the sound turned all the way down. See how much you can understand.

In 1993, a law was passed declaring that companies that make televisions bigger than 13 inches must build in decoders. This means that if you have a television that was made after 1993, you can see captions too. Many people who do not have hearing impairments like to watch television with the captions turned on because it helps them to improve their reading skills and helps them to understand what is happening on a television program better.

Bridges Beyond Sound
© 1996 Corinne K. Jensema
Paul H. Brookes Publishing Co., Inc.

S-11

Connect-the-Dots

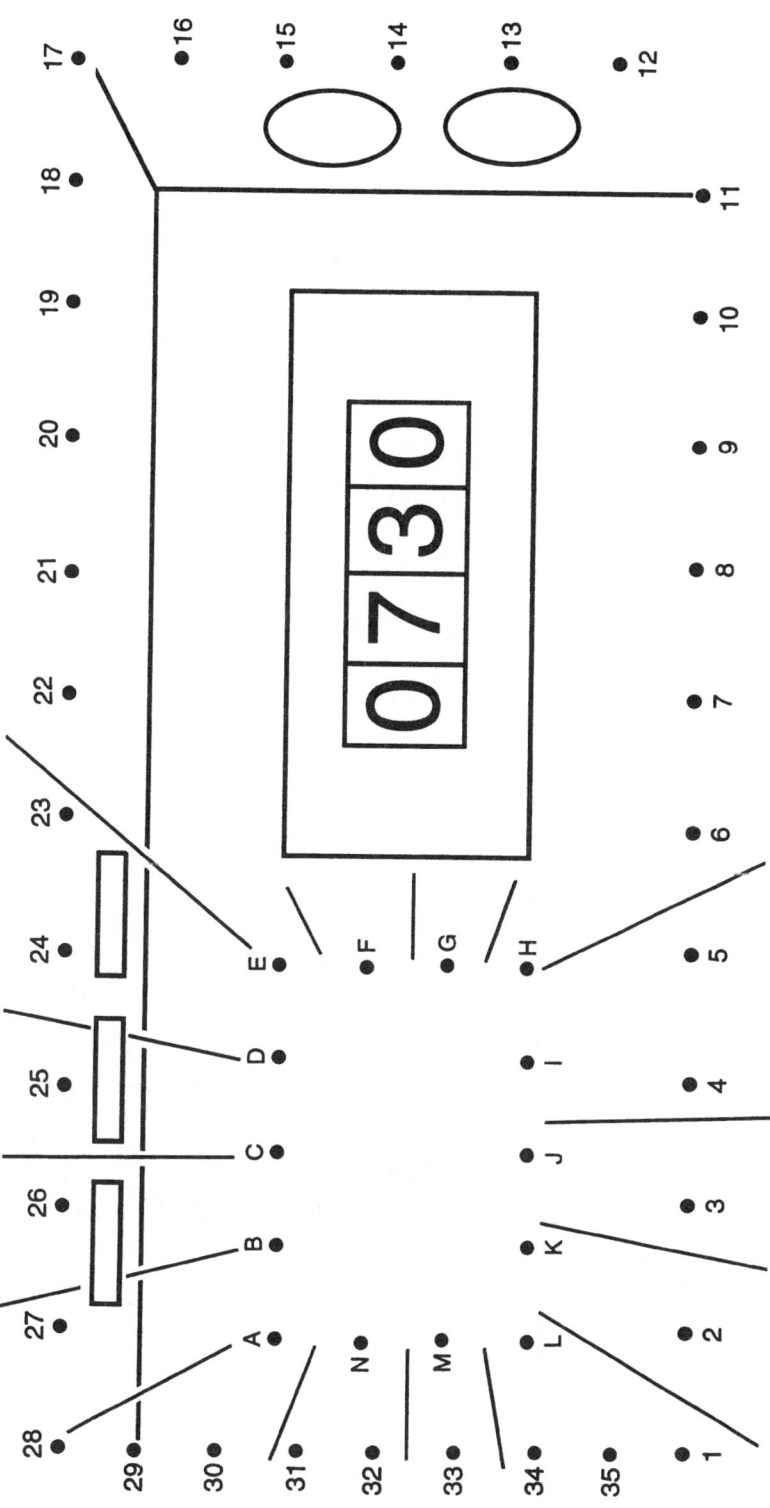

Bridges Beyond Sound
© 1996 Corinne K. Jensema
Paul H. Brookes Publishing Co., Inc.

S-11

CONNECT-THE-DOTS

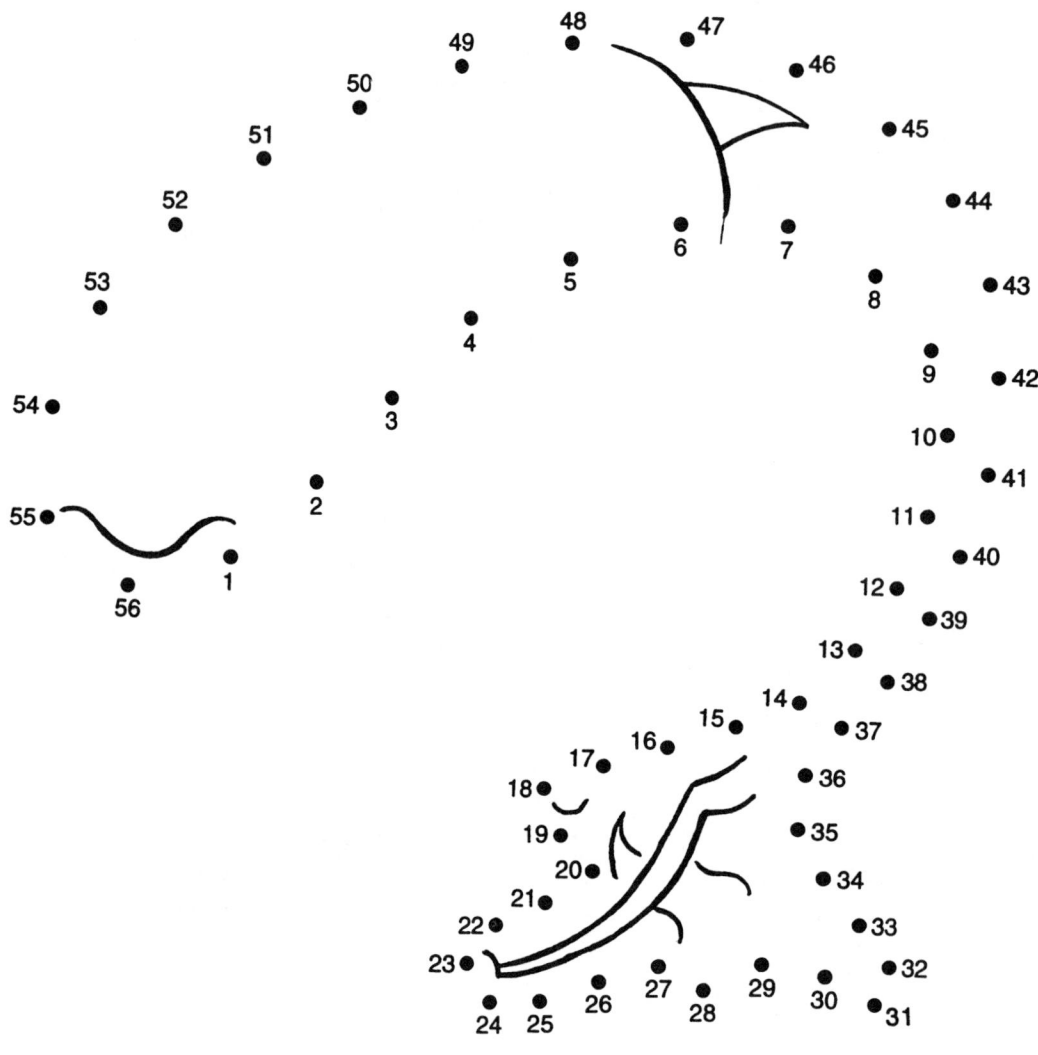

S-11

Connect-the-Dots

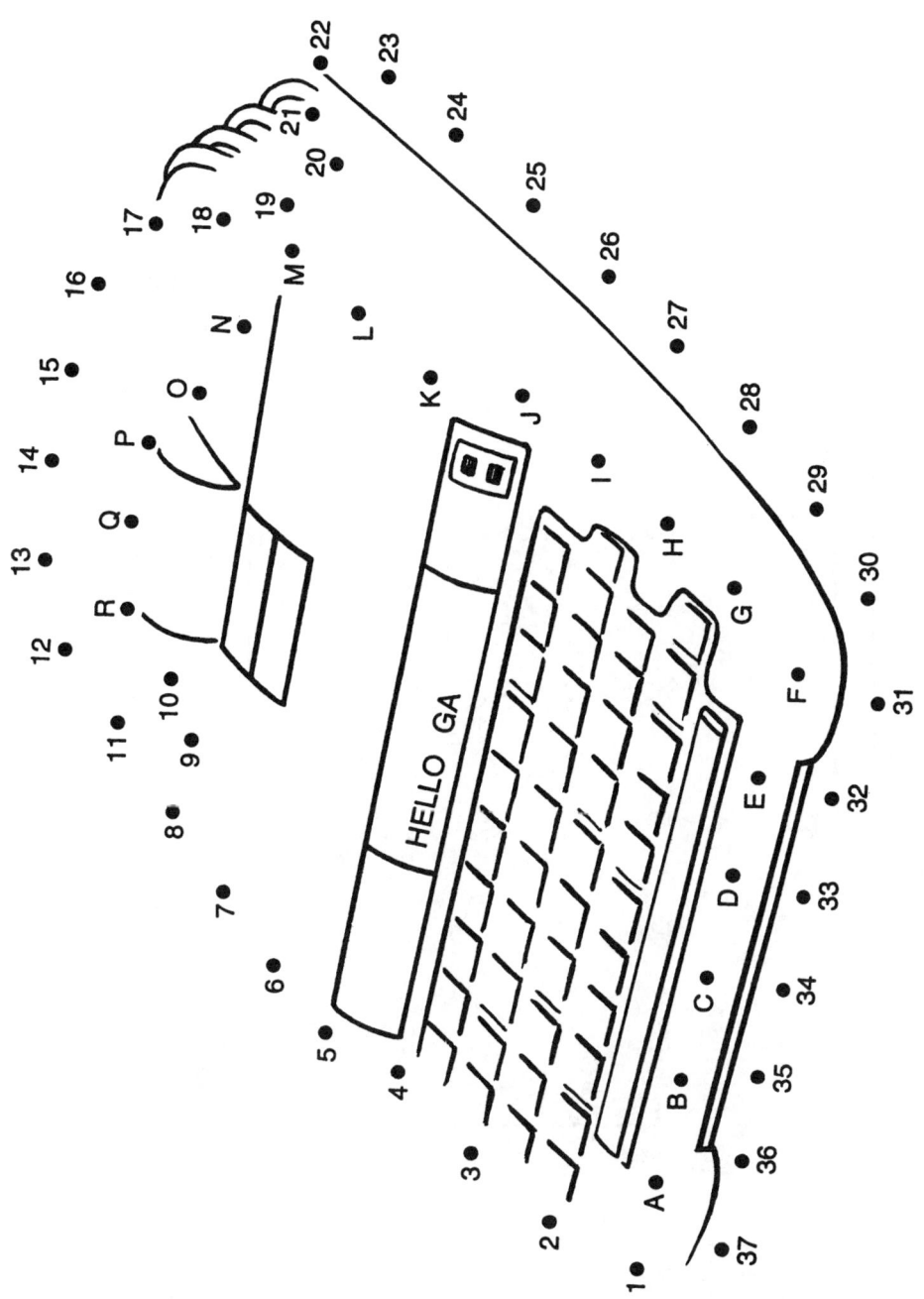

Bridges Beyond Sound
© 1996 Corinne K. Jensema
Paul H. Brookes Publishing Co., Inc.

S-11

CONNECT-THE-DOTS

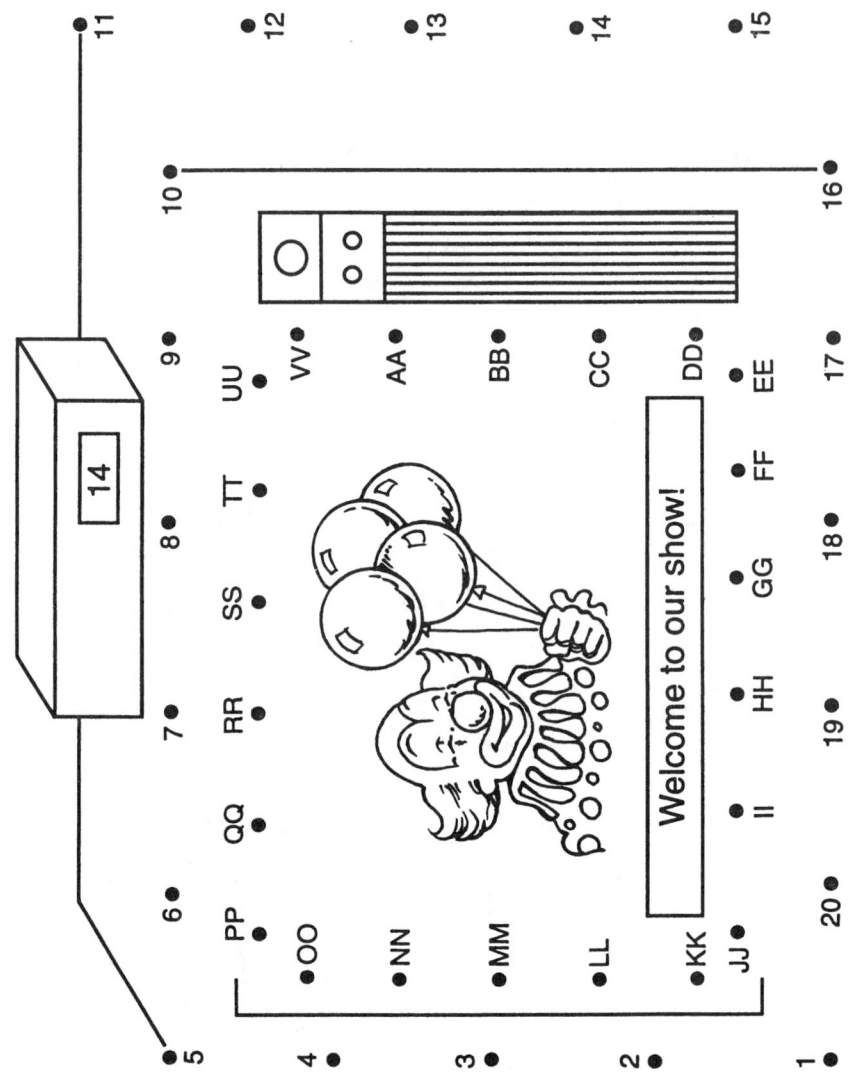

Bridges Beyond Sound
© 1996 Corinne K. Jensema
Paul H. Brookes Publishing Co., Inc.

S-12

WORD JUMBLE

Unscramble the letters for each item below to spell out different kinds of technologies used by people with hearing impairments.

1. slodec depcaonti veltsoenii

   _ _ _ _ _ _ - _ _ _ _ _ _ _ _ _   _ _ _ _ _ _ _ _ _ _
                   1

2. reddeoc

   _ _ _ _ _ _ _

3. henbid eht are grheina ida

   _ _ _ _ _ - _ _ _ - _ _ _   _ _ _ _ _ _ _   _ _ _
     2   3   4

4. gralinte svedcie

   _ _ _ _ _ _ _ _   _ _ _ _ _ _ _

5. ctmmaonitecleunio ecived rof het feda

   _ _ _ _ _ _ _ _ _ _ _ _ _ _ _ _ _   _ _ _ _ _ _   _ _ _
                   5

   _ _ _   _ _ _ _

6. ybod inharge ida

   _ _ _ _   _ _ _ _ _ _ _   _ _ _
      6

7. aybb ycr retdecot

   _ _ _ _   _ _ _   _ _ _ _ _ _ _ _
                    7

8. ni het rea rihnega dia

   _ _ - _ _ _ - _ _ _ _   _ _ _ _ _ _ _   _ _ _

9. mlaar kcolc

   _ _ _ _ _   _ _ _ _ _
    8

Bridges Beyond Sound
© 1996 Corinne K. Jensema
Paul H. Brookes Publishing Co., Inc.

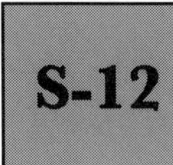

10. shlfgnia ghtli orf petonlehe

___ ___ ___ ___ ___ ___ ___ ___   ___ ___ ___ ___ ___   ___ ___ ___   ___ ___ ___ ___ ___ ___ ___ ___ ___ ___
                                                                                                                                         9

Now, take the numbered letters and put them in the spaces below to answer this question:

What feature of football was invented and first used at Gallaudet University, the only college for the deaf in the world?

___ ___ ___   ___ ___ ___ ___ ___ ___
 1 2 3   4 5 6 7 8 9

_____ _____ was invented at Gallaudet University by deaf football players to prevent the other teams from seeing and reading their signs when they would decide what play they were going to run. It is still used today for players to discuss what play to run and to exchange information without the other team being able to figure out what they are talking about.

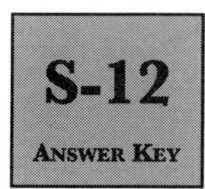

ANSWER KEY

WORD JUMBLE

Below are the answers to the word jumble worksheet.

1. slodec depcaonti veltsoenii   closed-cap<u>t</u>ioned television
2. reddeoc   <u>d</u>ecoder
3. henbid eht are grheina ida   be<u>h</u>ind-th<u>e</u>-ear <u>h</u>earing aid
4. gralinte svedcie   <u>a</u>lerting devices
5. ctmmaonitecleunio ecived rof het feda   telecomm<u>u</u>nication device for the deaf
6. ybod inharge ida   bo<u>d</u>y hearing aid
7. aybb ycr retdecot   baby cry <u>d</u>etector
8. ni het rea rihnega dia   in-the-ear hearing aid
9. mlaar kcolc   a<u>l</u>arm clock
10. shlfgnia ghtli orf petonlehe   flashing light for telephon<u>e</u>

What feature of football was invented and first used at Gallaudet University, the only college for the deaf in the world? <u>THE HUDDLE</u>

THE HUDDLE was invented at Gallaudet University by deaf football players to prevent the other teams from seeing and reading their signs when they would decide what play they were going to run. It is still used today for players to discuss what play to run and to exchange information without the other team being able to figure out what they are talking about.

Bridges Beyond Sound
© 1996 Corinne K. Jensema
Paul H. Brookes Publishing Co., Inc.

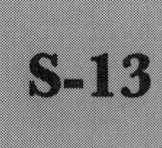

Communication Tips

WHEN SPEAKING AND SPEECHREADING

- Face the person who is deaf.
- Maintain eye contact with the person who is deaf.
- Be sure that there is a light source in front of you, not behind you.
- Speak more slowly than normal and try to be clear.
- Do not exaggerate your mouth movements.
- Keep objects and your hands away from your mouth.
- Isolate or emphasize key words.
- Give the person who is deaf as many visual cues as possible.
- Think about your words—some are easier to speechread than others.

WHEN WRITING AND/OR DRAWING

- Keep your writing to the point.
- Look for meaning, not grammar or spelling, in the message from the person who is deaf.
- When appropriate, use drawings in addition to your writing.

WHEN USING AN INTERPRETER

- Stand or sit next to the interpreter.
- Speak directly to the person who is deaf. Do not say to the interpreter, "Tell him [or her]...."
- Talk at a normal pace.
- Maintain eye contact with the person who is deaf.
- Allow time for the person who is deaf to ask and respond to questions.
- Remember that it is the interpreter's job to interpret *everything* you say; say only what you want interpreted.

Bridges Beyond Sound
© 1996 Corinne K. Jensema
Paul H. Brookes Publishing Co., Inc.

S-14

**INFORMATION SHEET ON
AMERICAN SIGN LANGUAGE**

American Sign Language (ASL) is the language used by the majority of people who are deaf or hard of hearing in the United States and who use a manual system of communication. In ASL, head, hand, and body movements, together with facial expressions, take the place of spoken words. Sign language is more complicated than the everyday gestures people who can hear use in conversation. In sign language, gestures are symbols that are made according to language rules. Each individual gesture is called a **sign.**

Each sign is made up of the following four components:

- Hand shape
- Hand position
- Direction of hand movement
- Palm orientation

The ways in which ASL signs can be combined are unique to this language. These combinations are not based on English or any other spoken language. Rather, ASL is put together to tell a message as the eye would see it. It "paints" a picture in a person's mind of the message being communicated.

How hard the sign is made (intensity) and how often it is repeated, along with facial expressions, are part of the meaning of ASL. By increasing the intensity and changing the facial expression accompanying a sign, the message can change from situation to situation.

Like English and other languages, ASL has regional dialects. The sign a person uses for a particular word may change depending on where in the United States the person has lived. This happens in English, too. For example, to describe a submarine sandwich, people in different parts of the United States use the word "sub," "hero," "hoagie," or "grinder." Also, just as each country around the world has its own spoken language, most have their own sign language as well.

Most people who can hear find it difficult to learn ASL. In ASL, words are not signed in the same order as a person would say them. For example, in English a person would say "There is a boy in the house," whereas it would be signed "House boy there inside."

Hearing people most often use a form of sign language called *Pidgin Signed English* (PSE). PSE uses the signs of ASL, but it follows English grammar. The purpose of PSE is to make it easier for people with and without hearing impairments to communicate with each other. Although PSE has no specific set of language rules, there are some general ones. Often, both people with and without

Bridges Beyond Sound
© 1996 Corinne K. Jensema
Paul H. Brookes Publishing Co., Inc.

S-14

hearing impairments will speak when using PSE. This allows both people to communicate using speechreading skills to understand the speaker's message. PSE is often used instead of ASL when a person with a hearing impairment is using his or her voice, because PSE follows English word order and ASL does not.

Fingerspelling is a hand (manual) representation of the 26 letters of the English alphabet. Fingerspelling is used in sign language when an English word has no sign for it. The most frequently fingerspelled words are names for people, places, and things, as well as highly technical words. Fingerspelling is used in all sign communication systems, but more often in those that follow English word order and grammar.

When a person is fingerspelling, the palm of his or her hand should face the person who is receiving the message. Each letter should be made clearly, with a slight pause between words. The arm should be kept still while spelling. The person fingerspelling should be able to see the back of his or her own hand when fingerspelling.

SUGGESTED READINGS

DiPietro, L. (1981). *A look at American Sign Language.* Washington, DC: The National Academy of Gallaudet University.
DiPietro, L. (1982). *A look at fingerspelling.* Washington, DC: The National Academy of Gallaudet University.
Shroyer, E.H. (1982). *Signs of the times.* Washington, DC: Gallaudet University Press.

S-15

AMERICAN MANUAL ALPHABET

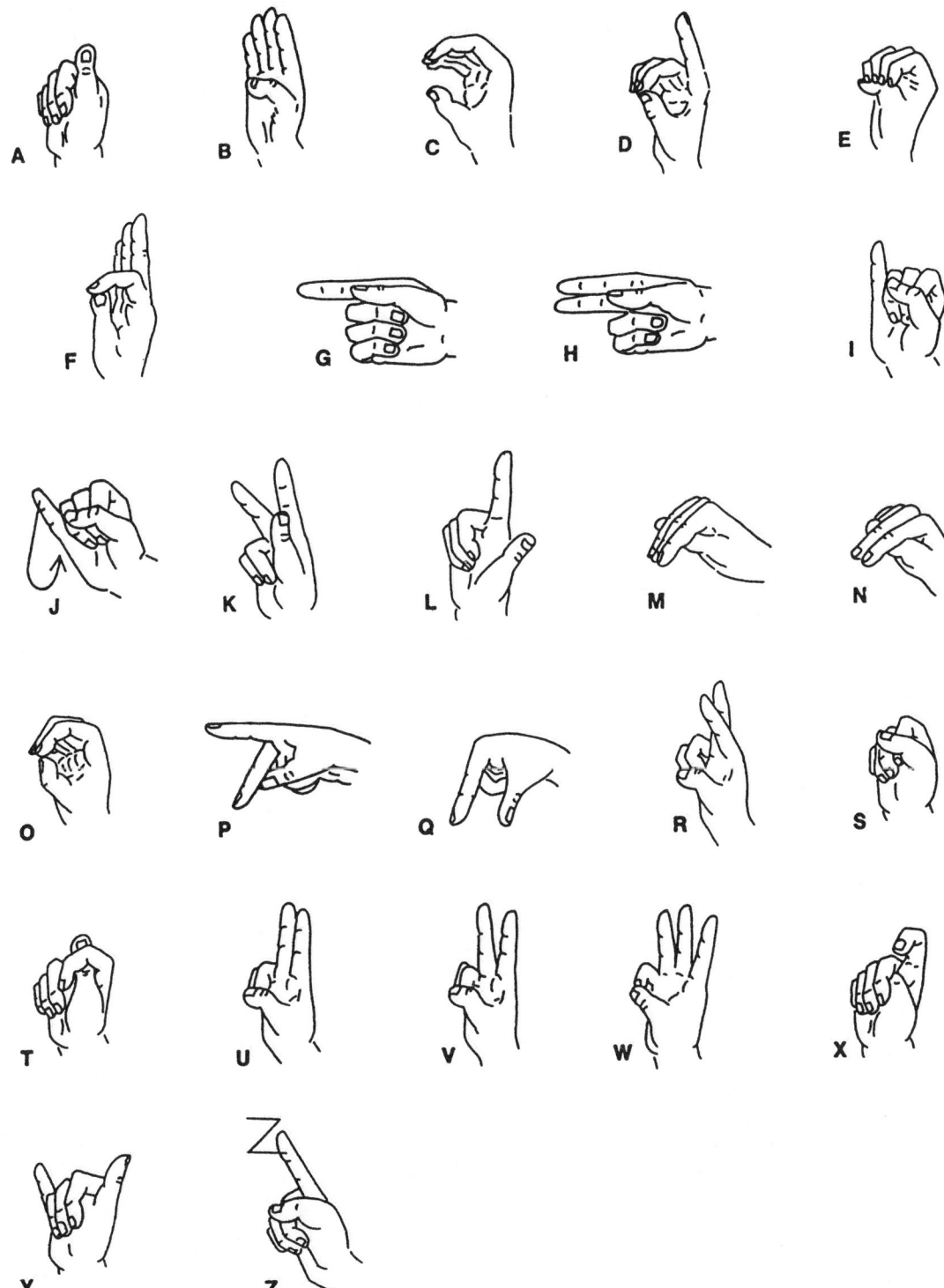

From Riekenof, L. (1987). *The joy of signing* (2nd ed.). Springfield, MO: Gospel Publishing House; reprinted by permission.

S-16

FINGERSPELLING

Fingerspelling is the way people with hearing impairments say the alphabet. Each letter has a specific hand shape. You might have seen this kind of spelling on *Sesame Street* or in books. Use the chart (S-15) to practice how each letter is made. When your teacher tells you, pick a partner and spell the sentences below to each other.

1. My name is _____ .

2. My address is _____ .

3. My favorite food is _____ .

4. I like to play _____ .

5. I have a _____ .

6. The name of my school is _____ .

Bridges Beyond Sound
© 1996 Corinne K. Jensema
Paul H. Brookes Publishing Co., Inc.

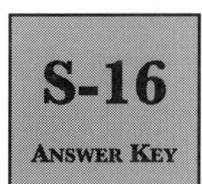

FINGERSPELLING

Have students read the explanation of American Sign Language (S-14) and the American Manual Alphabet (S-15) and review and practice each letter on the fingerspelling chart. Each student should then select a partner and fingerspell each of the sentences below to each other.

1. My name is _____ .

2. My address is _____ .

3. My favorite food is _____ .

4. I like to play _____ (sport, game, etc.).

5. I have a _____ (kind of pet—or if child does not have a pet, a favorite toy, etc.).

6. The name of my school is _____ .

Bridges Beyond Sound
© 1996 Corinne K. Jensema
Paul H. Brookes Publishing Co., Inc.

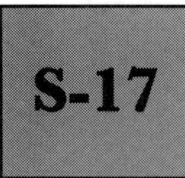

S-17

**CHILDREN'S BOOKS
ABOUT PEOPLE WHO ARE DEAF**

Adams, B. (1979). *Like it is: Facts and feelings about handicaps from kids who know.* New York: Walder.
Aseltine, L. (1986). *I'm deaf and it's okay.* Niles, IL: A. Whitman & Co.
Bergman, T. (1989). *Finding a common language.* Milwaukee, WI: Gareth Stevens Publishing.
Bove, L. (1980). *Sesame Street sign language fun.* New York: Random House.
Carroll, C. (1991). *Laurent Clerc: The story of his early years.* Washington, DC: Kendall Green Publications.
Corcoran, B. (1974). *A dance to still music.* New York: Atheneum.
Curtis, P. (1981). *Cindy, a hearing ear dog.* New York: Dutton.
Ferrigno, L. (1982). *The incredible Lou Ferrigno: His story.* New York: Simon & Schuster.
Glazzard, M.H. (1978). *Meet Camille and Danielle: They are special persons.* Lawrence, KS: H & H Enterprises, Inc.
Goldfeder, C., & Goldfeder, J. (1973). *The girl who wouldn't talk.* Silver Spring, MD: National Association of the Deaf.
Greenberg, J.E. (1985). *What is the sign for friend?* New York: F. Watts.
Greene, L. (1981). *Sign language.* New York: F. Watts.
Greene, L. (1990). *Sign me fine: Experiencing American Sign Language.* Washington, DC: Kendall Green Publications.
Hanlon, E. (1979). *The swing.* Scarsdale, NY: Bradbury Press.
Hirsch, K. (1981). *Becky.* Minneapolis: Carolrhoda Books.
Hunter, E.F. (1963). *Child of the silent night.* Boston: Houghton Mifflin.
Hyman, J. (1980). *Deafness.* New York: F. Watts.
Ireland, K. (1980). *Kitty O'Neil: Daredevil woman.* New York: Harvey House.
Keller, H. (1974). *Story of my life.* West Haven, CT: Pendulum Press.
Lee, J.M. (1991). *Silent lotus.* New York: Farrar, Straus & Giroux.
Levine, E.S. (1974). *Lisa and her soundless world.* New York: Human Sciences Press.
Lewis, C.C. (1991). *Hello, Alexander Graham Bell speaking: A biography.* New York: Dillon Press.
Neimark, A.E. (1983). *A deaf child listened: Thomas Gallaudet, pioneer in American education.* New York: Morrow.
Peter, D. (1976). *Claire and Emma.* London: A & C Black.
Peterson, J.W. (1977). *I have a sister—My sister is deaf.* New York: Harper & Row.
Rennei, E.C. (1965). *Tim and his hearing aid.* Washington, DC: Alexander Graham Bell Association for the Deaf.
Riskind, M. (1981). *Apple is my sign.* Boston: Houghton Mifflin.
Robinette, D. (1990). *Hometown heroes: Successful deaf youth in America.* Washington, DC: Kendall Green Publications.
Rosen, L. (1981). *Just like everybody else.* New York: Harcourt Brace Jovanovich.
St. George, J. (1992). *Dear Dr. Bell—Your friend, Helen Keller.* New York: Putnam's Sons.
Starowitz, A.M. (1988). *The day we met Cindy.* Washington, DC: Kendall Green Publications.

Bridges Beyond Sound
© 1996 Corinne K. Jensema
Paul H. Brookes Publishing Co., Inc.

S-17

Thacher, A.M. (1980). *Fastest woman on earth*. Milwaukee, WI: Raintree Publishers.
Toole, D.K. (1980). *Courageous deaf adults*. Beaverton, OR: Dormac, Inc.
Toole, D.K. (1981). *Successful deaf Americans*. Beaverton, OR: Dormac, Inc.
Walker, L.A. (1985). *Amy: The story of a deaf child*. New York: E.P. Dutton.
Wolf, B. (1977). *Anna's silent world*. Philadelphia: J.B. Lippincott.

S-18

HISTORY OF DEAF PEOPLE IN THE UNITED STATES

The first information about teaching deaf children in the United States can be found in a book, written in 1793, by Dr. William Thornton. He was the first person to head the U.S. Patent Office and he also designed the U.S. Capitol building.

In 1803, 10 years later, Francis Green, the father of a boy who was deaf, counted the number of deaf people in Massachusetts—there were 70 people. He guessed that there were 500 deaf people in the United States. (In 1994, there were 2–3 million deaf people in the United States.) Francis Green sent his son, Charles, to a school for the deaf in Edinburgh, Scotland, run by Thomas Braidwood. Charles Green became the first U.S. citizen who was deaf to get an education.

In 1813, Colonel William Bolling of Virginia learned that John Braidwood, grandson of Thomas Braidwood, was living in Baltimore. Colonel Bolling had two deaf brothers, one deaf sister, and two deaf children, William and Mary. He gave Braidwood the job of teaching his children. William and Mary became the first deaf children to get an education in the United States. John Braidwood tried to start schools in both Baltimore and New York, but he had no luck. He started one in Cobbs, Virginia, in 1815, but it failed because he did not always show up for work.

One of the most widely known stories about educating deaf children in the United States began in 1814. Thomas Hopkins Gallaudet was watching his younger brothers and sisters play with some other children. One of the children, Alice Cogswell, was not playing with the other children. He found out she was deaf. He taught her the word for "hat" by pointing to his own hat and writing the word with a stick in the sand. When Alice's father, Dr. Mason Cogswell, learned about the writing lesson, he was very happy. Dr. Cogswell talked to Thomas Gallaudet about starting a school for the deaf in the United States.

Dr. Cogswell paid for Thomas Gallaudet to go to Europe and find out how deaf people were educated there. In Paris, he found the Institution for the Education of the Deaf and Dumb. This school had been founded in 1755 and was the first free school for the deaf in the world. Thomas Gallaudet met a deaf teacher there named Laurent Clerc. Laurent Clerc agreed to come to the United States to be the first deaf person in the country to teach the deaf. Thomas Gallaudet and Laurent Clerc took a boat from France to the United States. While on the long trip across the Atlantic Ocean, Laurent Clerc learned English by writing in a diary and having Thomas Gallaudet correct his writing. Thomas Gallaudet learned sign language from Laurent Clerc. This is why the sign language used in the United States has its roots in French sign language.

Bridges Beyond Sound
© 1996 Corinne K. Jensema
Paul H. Brookes Publishing Co., Inc.

S-18

Thomas Gallaudet and Laurent Clerc opened the first permanent school for the deaf, the Connecticut Asylum for the Education and Instruction of Deaf and Dumb Persons, in 1817. It cost $200 a year to live at the school and attend classes there. Within a few years, there were other schools for the deaf in New York City, Philadelphia, and Danville, Kentucky.

In 1836, Samuel F.B. Morse invented the telegraph. This fact later led to the founding of Gallaudet University, the only university for the deaf in the world, located in Washington, D.C. Morse was married to a deaf woman. He spoke to her by tapping his fingers on her hands. Morse hired Amos Kendall to be his money manager. Morse strung his first telegraph line between the Library of Congress in Washington, D.C., and Baltimore, Maryland. The line went through Kendall's land. Morse's famous words, "What hath God wrought?", were sent over this line. Both men became rich from the telegraph. Kendall gave his land for the building of the Columbia Institution for the Instruction of the Deaf and Dumb and Blind. President Abraham Lincoln signed the charter allowing the college to be built. The college was then renamed the National Deaf-Mute College. In 1884 it was renamed Gallaudet College and then Gallaudet University in 1986. The President of the United States still signs the diplomas of all of Gallaudet University's graduates.

A man named Bernard Engelsman came to New York from Mr. Deutsch's Jewish School in Vienna, Austria, 2 months after the founding of the National Deaf-Mute College. He began a small school using the *German method*, which used speech and no sign language. This became known as the *oral method*. His school later became the Lexington School for the Deaf, which still teaches deaf children today. Bringing the oral method to the United States started a disagreement that people still argue about, concerning whether it is better to teach children who are deaf with signs or orally.

In 1864, Gardiner G. Hubbard, whose deaf daughter later married Alexander Graham Bell, asked the Massachusetts legislature to give money for a school to teach the oral method to deaf people. The American Asylum, the school for the deaf in Massachusetts, was against the oral method because its staff believed it was not a good idea. They believed that deaf people learned more effectively through sign language. It was decided by the Massachusetts legislature that the method had to be tried more before any money would be given to an oral school. Mr. Hubbard started a school on his own with a teacher named Harriet Rogers. He tried to get important people to agree with his beliefs. One of these important people, John Clarke, gave the state $50,000 to start a school in Northampton. This school became the Clarke School for the Deaf, which still uses the oral method today.

Bridges Beyond Sound
© 1996 Corinne K. Jensema
Paul H. Brookes Publishing Co., Inc.

S-18

After the Civil War, schools for African American children who were deaf started forming. North Carolina was the first state to open a school for deaf African American children.

The first school in which deaf children were included in general classes was a private school in Baltimore, Maryland, opened by Frederick Knapp in 1877. Knapp's school taught German. About 100 of the 17,000 children who were taught there were deaf. Hearing children were not allowed to sign to the deaf children. If any children signed, they had to wear gloves for punishment. In the late-1800s, many of the schools that used sign language began using the oral method.

Just before the Civil War, several state associations of the deaf were formed. An *association* is a group of people who meet for a good cause. A meeting was held in 1850 in Hartford, Connecticut, in Thomas Gallaudet's and Laurent Clerc's honor. During the meeting, a national association of the deaf was suggested. Deaf people felt it was important to meet because the oral method was taking over and deaf teachers were no longer getting jobs. In 1853, a national association was founded. Edwin A. Hodgson is considered the father and founder of the National Association of the Deaf.

At the same time that the National Association of the Deaf was being formed, hearing teachers of the deaf from all over the world met in Milan, Italy. The educators of the deaf at this meeting voted to ban sign language from being taught to deaf children. The Americans at the meeting were against the ban. They believed that sign language and speech should be used together.

Dr. Alexander Graham Bell, inventor of the telephone, was interested in deafness because his wife was deaf. He felt that deaf people should not be allowed to marry other deaf people because he thought this would cause more deaf children to be born. He thought that deaf people should not be encouraged to get together for fun, business, or religious reasons. He thought that schools should not hire deaf teachers. Because he was so widely known, many people believed him. Edward Allen Fay, editor of the *American Annals of the Deaf*, a widely known magazine about deaf research, wrote a major report to give a different opinion because many people who were deaf were afraid other people would believe Bell.

Bell was awarded the Volta Prize for his invention of the telephone. He used the money to set up a center in Washington, D.C., to house information about deafness. The building was called the Volta Bureau. This library is still one of the world's best for information about deafness.

In the 1890s, people became aware that students who were deaf needed to be taught a trade. Trade classes were added at some schools for the deaf and at

Bridges Beyond Sound
© 1996 Corinne K. Jensema
Paul H. Brookes Publishing Co., Inc.

S-18

the National Deaf-Mute College. Many people who were deaf received training as printers.

Getting insurance was always a problem for deaf people. In 1898, a group of young deaf men met at the Michigan School for the Deaf and began the Fraternal Society of the Deaf, an insurance company for the deaf. When the company first began, it offered policies to cover funeral expenses, but later added policies for sickness and accidents as well.

Because more deaf people were beginning to get an education, they also were beginning to get better jobs. They became nurses, inventors, artists, and shop keepers. One deaf inventor, John R. Gregg, invented Gregg Shorthand, a way to use fewer pencil marks to speed up writing, which is still used today. Deaf people were also becoming more active in sports. Schools for the deaf started having baseball, football, and wrestling teams. William Hoy was a famous deaf baseball player for the Cincinnati Reds and Washington Senators. He invented the hand count in baseball because he could not hear what the umpire was saying. Paul Hubbard, a quarterback on Gallaudet's football team from 1893 to 1895, said he invented the huddle so that the other team could not read the deaf players' sign language. In 1916, a group of deaf men put together a semiprofessional football team called the Goodyear Silents because many of them worked near or at the Goodyear rubber plants. They won the Central Ohio Championship and were undefeated in 1918. They even won with a score of 115–0 against a Canadian team that was undefeated.

Several important events that affected deaf people occurred during and after World War II. In 1954, the Supreme Court outlawed separate schools for Caucasian and African American deaf children. In 1958, President Eisenhower signed a law to set up Captioned Films for the Deaf. This program put words or subtitles on movies so that deaf people could understand what was being said in the movies. These movies are lent to schools and clubs for the deaf. The Registry of Interpreters for the Deaf (RID) was started in 1964. RID represents people who work as sign language interpreters for people who are deaf. They work to make interpreting a more professional job. Among its members are sign language and oral interpreters, and RID tests these interpreters to make sure they can do a good job. The National Theater of the Deaf, a company of deaf and hearing actors who perform plays in sign language, was started in 1966 and did its first tour the next year. Deaf students received a better chance to get good job training education when the National Technical Institute for the Deaf was set up on the college campus of the Rochester Institute of Technology in New York. In 1975, PL 94-142, the Education for All Handicapped Children Act, was passed by Congress and promised that all children with disabilities could get a free and appropriate public education in the United States. An important part of this law was

Bridges Beyond Sound
© 1996 Corinne K. Jensema
Paul H. Brookes Publishing Co., Inc.

that schools now had to try to make special education possible in children's home schools.

There was a lot of progress made in technology after 1960. Before 1964, deaf people could not use the regular telephone. In 1964, Robert Weitbrecht invented a machine called a teletypewriter (TTY) that allowed deaf people to type to each other over the telephone instead of using their voices. TTYs later became known as telecommunication devices for the deaf (TDDs). In 1990, two important laws were passed by Congress. PL 101-336, the Americans with Disabilities Act (ADA) of 1990, forced states to have relay operators who could interpret TTY typing to speaking so that deaf and hearing people could talk to each other over the telephone. PL 101-431, the Television Decoder Circuitry Act, forced television makers to put devices (decoders) in their television sets so that people can have words or closed captions appear on their television screens. Today if you buy a television with a screen that is 13 inches or bigger, it will have a button on it that will let you see the closed captions.

One of the most important events to take place in the history of deaf people in the United States was a protest by the students of Gallaudet College (presently known as Gallaudet University) in 1988. The students did not want the president of the university to be a hearing person. They forced the university to tell the hearing person they picked for the job that she could not keep it. They picked Dr. I. King Jordan, a deaf professor at the university, to be the first deaf president of Gallaudet.

REFERENCES

American with Disabilities Act (ADA) of 1990, PL 101-336. (July 26, 1990). Title 42, U.S.C. 12101 et seq: *U.S. Statutes at Large, 104,* 327–378.

Education for All Handicapped Children Act of 1975, PL 94-142. (August 23, 1977). Title 20, U.S.C. 1401 et seq: *U.S. Statutes at Large, 89,* 773–796.

Television Decoder Circuitry Act of 1990, PL 101-431. (October 15, 1990). Title 47, U.S.C. 303 & 330 et seq: *U.S. Statutes at Large,* 104, 960–961.

Bridges Beyond Sound
© 1996 Corinne K. Jensema
Paul H. Brookes Publishing Co., Inc.

S-19

SUCCESSFUL PEOPLE WITH HEARING IMPAIRMENTS

There have been many people with hearing impairments who have made important contributions to a variety of fields throughout history. Below are brief biographical sketches of a few successful people with hearing impairments.

KATHY BUCKLEY

Kathy Buckley is a professional stand-up comedienne. She performs in nightclubs and comedy clubs all over the United States. She is billed as the first comedienne with a hearing impairment to perform for hearing audiences. Buckley was honored with a nomination for "Best Female Stand-Up Comedienne" during the American Comedy Awards.

Buckley grew up in Ohio. She is not sure whether she was born with a hearing impairment or lost her hearing when she became ill with meningitis when she was 4 years old. Her family did not know Kathy had a hearing loss until she was in second grade. She had been identified as a slow learner and placed in a school for children with mental retardation. Later, her hearing loss was discovered and she returned to public school.

In her late teens, Buckley's life was interrupted when she was run over by a jeep while sunbathing on a beach. This accident caused paralysis, which came and went for 5 years. Six years after the accident, she developed cervical cancer. Undaunted, Buckley has turned roadblocks into springboards, using her personal experiences as a launching pad for humor and education.

Her first experience as a comedienne occurred when, on a dare from a friend, she entered a comedy contest, "Stand-up Comics Take a Stand," in 1988. Buckley easily won fourth place and soon began touring the country, playing major comedy venues. In a remarkably short time, she made her mark as an extremely popular comic with materials based on, among other things, her hearing loss.

ERASTUS "DEAF" SMITH

Erastus "Deaf" Smith was a soldier in the Texas army during the Mexican War. He served as a scout and guide under General Stephen Austin. Smith's hearing impairment began at birth and was complicated by many serious illnesses.

Smith was born in New York in 1787, grew up in Mississippi, and moved to Texas in 1821. When he was asked if his hearing impairment was a problem he replied, "No, I sometimes think it is an advantage. I have learned to keep a sharp outlook and I am never disturbed by the whistling of a ball [bullet]. I don't hear the bark till I feel the bite." In the Battle of San Jacinto, Deaf Smith devised a plan to cut off the Texans and the Mexicans from retreat, which forced them to fight

Bridges Beyond Sound
© 1996 Corinne K. Jensema
Paul H. Brookes Publishing Co., Inc.

to the finish. The Texans overpowered the more numerous Mexicans and captured their general. Texas won its independence and Smith became a folk hero. A Northern Texas county was named Deaf Smith County. National brands of peanut butter, and pancake, waffle, and biscuit mix were named after him. Smith's picture appeared on the $5 bill issued by the Republic of Texas.

Erastus "Deaf" Smith died on November 30, 1837, while scouting in Texas. He is buried in Richmond, Texas. The inscription on his tombstone reads, "So valiant and trustworthy was he that all titles sink into insignificance before the simple name of 'Deaf' Smith."

LAURENT CLERC

Laurent Clerc, a deaf teacher, taught at the National Royal Institution of the Deaf in Paris. Clerc agreed to come to the United States with Thomas Gallaudet and open America's first school for the deaf—The American School for the Deaf, in Hartford, Connecticut. Clerc was America's first deaf teacher of the deaf and four of his students became teachers of the deaf. Both Gallaudet and Clerc spent their lives working to educate deaf people. Efforts are being made to establish a Laurent Clerc Day to be celebrated annually in schools and in the deaf community.

ROBERT DAVILA

Dr. Robert Davila was appointed by former President George Bush as the Assistant Secretary for the Office of Special Education and Rehabilitative Services at the U.S. Department of Education. At the time, he was the highest ranking federal officer who had a hearing impairment. Davila was born in July 1932. He was one of eight children of a migrant family of farm workers who immigrated to the United States from Mexico. Davila lost his hearing from meningitis as a young boy.

Davila earned several degrees, including a Bachelor of Arts degree in education of the hearing impaired, a Master of Science degree in special education, and a Doctor of Philosophy degree in educational technology. Before he became the Assistant Secretary, he was the Vice President of Pre-College Programs at Gallaudet University. After leaving his government job, he became Headmaster at the New York School for the Deaf in Rochester, New York.

LINDA BOVE

Linda Bove is an actress best known for her role on the children's television program *Sesame Street*. She has appeared on the soap opera *Search for Tomorrow*,

Bridges Beyond Sound
© 1996 Corinne K. Jensema
Paul H. Brookes Publishing Co., Inc.

played on Broadway, and acted in *Children of a Lesser God*. She also has directed plays in Connecticut and California.

Bove was born with a hearing impairment. She has been featured in *Sesame Street* books about sign language and appears around the country as a lecturer. She has received a number of awards for her contributions to the field of theater, including one by the Action for Children's Television and Parent's Choice Award for *Sign-Me-A-Story* and an honorary doctorate degree from Gallaudet University.

MARLEE MATLIN

Marlee Matlin is best known for her starring role in the film, *Children of a Lesser God*. She won an Academy Award for "Best Actress" for her role as the lead character in this movie. She is the youngest person to receive this award and only one of four people who ever received this award for their debut film. She is probably the best-known deaf actress in the United States. She has also starred in the series *Reasonable Doubts*, the movie *Hear No Evil*, and the television movie *Bridge to Silence,* and she has made guest appearances on other television programs, including *Seinfeld* and *Picket Fences.* She has appeared in music videos for Billy Joel and Garth Brooks. For Super Bowl XXVII, she signed the National Anthem while Garth Brooks sang.

Matlin lost her hearing when she was 18 months old. She was born and raised in Morton Grove, Illinois. She began her theatrical career at the age of 7 in the role of Dorothy in *The Wizard of Oz* at a children's theater company in Chicago.

Matlin is a strong advocate for the rights and needs of people who have hearing impairments. She is involved in many charities, particularly those that serve children. She is a national spokesperson for the National Captioning Institute, encouraging awareness and funding of closed captioning for television and videotapes.

LOUIS FRISINO

Louis Frisino is a widely known Maryland wildlife artist. Most of his works are watercolors. His paintings are realistic and very detailed.

Louis Frisino was born deaf in January 1934. He went to Xavier School for the Deaf and Maryland School for the Deaf. He studied art at the Maryland Institute College of Art. For 25 years, he was an artist for a newspaper, *The News American.* Now he has a private career as a wildlife artist. Two of his paintings were used by the National Wildlife Federation as Christmas cards. Frisino has

Bridges Beyond Sound
© 1996 Corinne K. Jensema
Paul H. Brookes Publishing Co., Inc.

won many contests for his artwork of ducks and other wildlife, including the Federal Duck Stamp Contest.

I. [IRVING] KING JORDAN

Dr. I. King Jordan is the first deaf president of Gallaudet University. He was selected after the students at Gallaudet staged a protest when Gallaudet University selected a hearing woman as the university's president. The students wanted a deaf president.

Jordan was born in June 1943. Not long after he finished his tour of duty in the U.S. Army, Jordan was in a motorcycle accident, which resulted in his profound hearing loss. After he recovered, he attended college and received a doctoral degree in psychology from the University of Tennessee. Jordan taught for many years at Galluadet University before becoming its president.

NELLIE WILLHITE

Nellie Willhite was the first woman in South Dakota, and perhaps the first deaf person in the world, to become a pilot. Her interest in flying was stimulated by Charles Lindberg's famous flight across the Atlantic Ocean in *The Spirit of St. Louis* in 1927. Willhite realized that there were two barriers to overcome to realize her dream of becoming a pilot: 1) female pilots were almost unheard of at that time, and 2) she was a deaf female pilot. Nevertheless, she enrolled in a pilot's course and after 13 hours of instruction she soloed in January 1928.

Her father gave her a plane as a gift and she became a barnstormer, flying in air shows and air races throughout the Midwest. Her stunts made her a folk hero in South Dakota. Willhite was also a member of the "Ninety Nines," a group of female pilots that was founded, in part, by Amelia Earhart.

DOUGLAS TILDEN

Douglas Tilden is one of California's most famous sculptors and the best-known deaf sculptor in the country. Tilden was born in May 1860, and lost his hearing when he was 4 years old from scarlet fever. He attended the California School for the Deaf and it was there that he was tutored by Theophilus d'Estrella, a deaf artist, photographer, and teacher. Tilden worked at the University of California as a teacher, and then left to attend the Academy of Design in New York. He later studied in Paris. Tilden's work can be found throughout the West Coast. Tilden died in his studio at the age of 75 in August 1935.

Bridges Beyond Sound
© 1996 Corinne K. Jensema
Paul H. Brookes Publishing Co., Inc.

S-19

JOHN CLARKE

John Clarke grew up in Glacier National Park in the Rocky Mountains of Montana where he loved wild animals and studied them in depth. He made figures out of clay and later began carving them from wood. As a young boy, he became deaf from scarlet fever.

Clarke was born in January 1881 to Native American parents in Montana. He attended the Montana and North Dakota Schools for the Deaf and studied wood carving at the St. Francis Academy in Milwaukee. Clarke was called "Catapuis" in his Native American language, which means "man-who-talks-not." Clarke opened a studio in Montana where he sold his carvings to tourists, including John D. Rockefeller.

His carvings are now on display at the Montana Historical Society Museum and at the University of Montana. Clarke died in November 1970 at the age of 89.

HEATHER WHITESTONE

Heather Whitestone was crowned Miss America on September 17, 1994. Whitestone has encouraged other people through her STARS program. STARS means "Success Through Action and Realization of Your Dreams." Her five-point STARS platform is dedicated to students with and without hearing impairments; it conveys the message that "Anything Is Possible."

Whitestone is 21 years old. She lost her hearing when she was 18 months old after receiving an inoculation that caused a high fever. The medication saved her life but caused deafness.

After her reign as Miss America, Whitestone returned to college to complete her studies. Her faithful platform will continue as always to encourage children to build their self-esteem and believe in themselves and their dreams.

Bridges Beyond Sound
© 1996 Corinne K. Jensema
Paul H. Brookes Publishing Co., Inc.

S-19

KATHY BUCKLEY

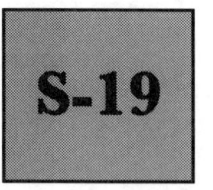

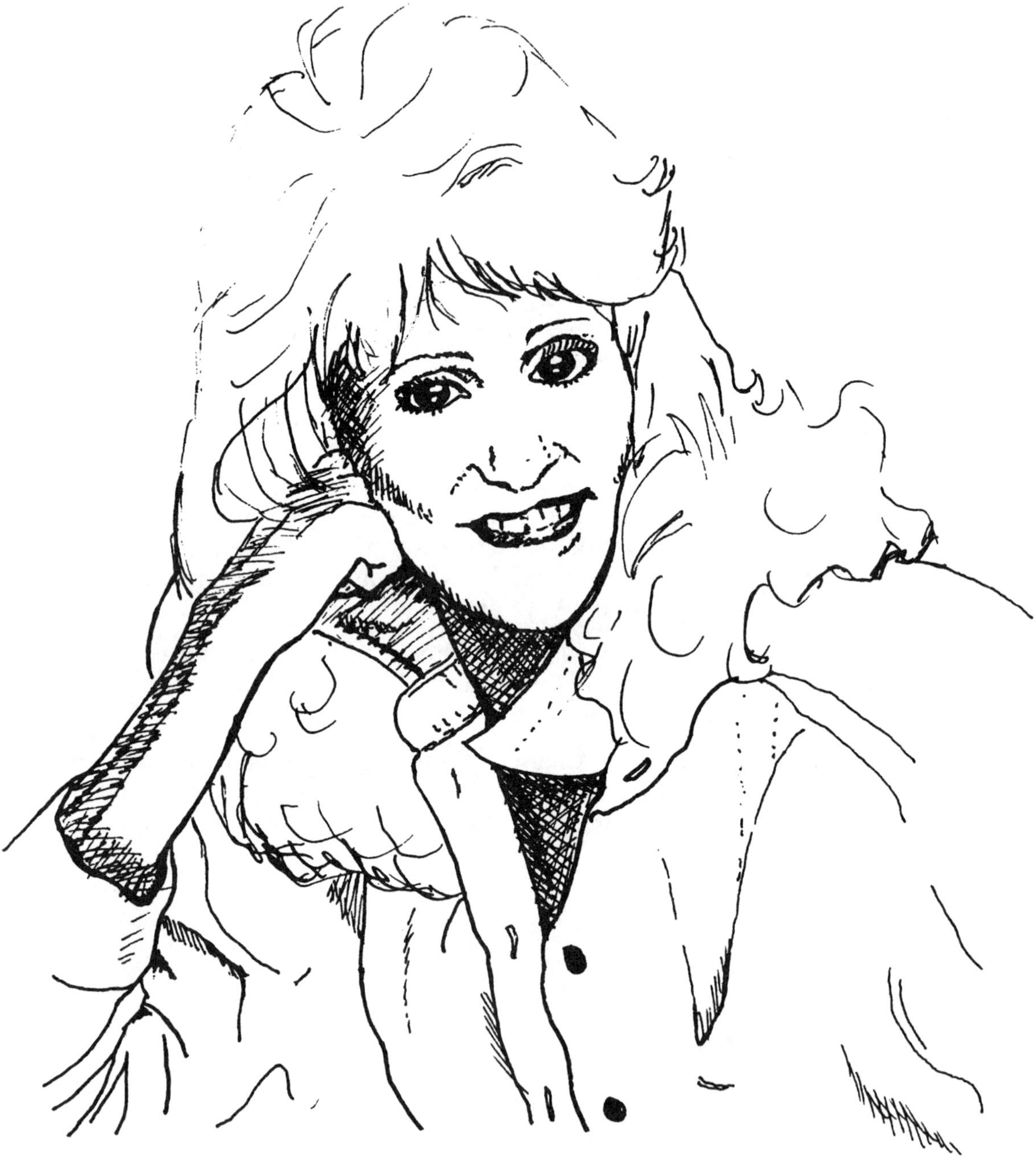

Bridges Beyond Sound
© 1996 Corinne K. Jensema
Paul H. Brookes Publishing Co., Inc.

S-19
Erastus "Deaf" Smith

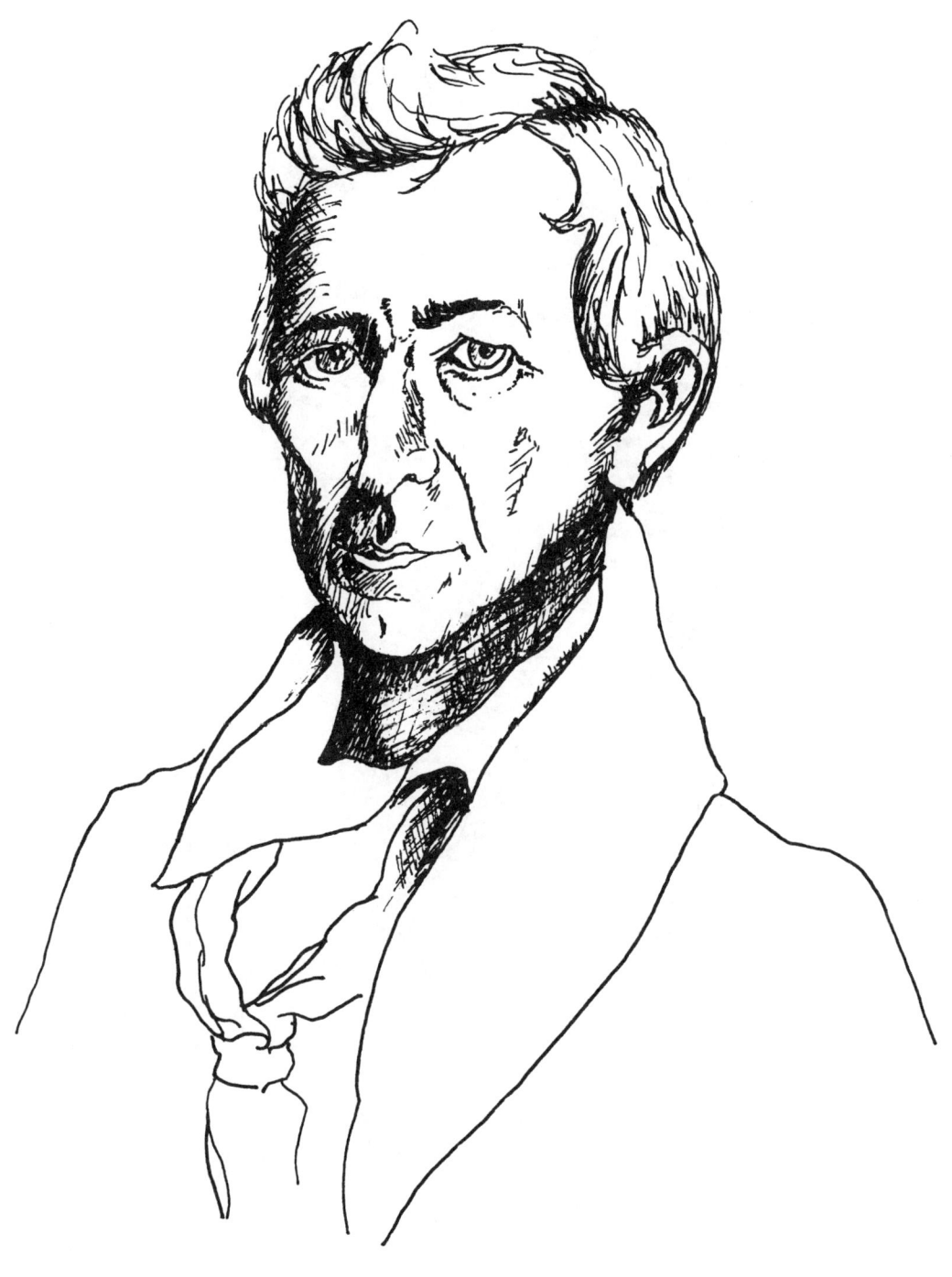

Bridges Beyond Sound
© 1996 Corinne K. Jensema
Paul H. Brookes Publishing Co., Inc.

S-19
LAURENT CLERC

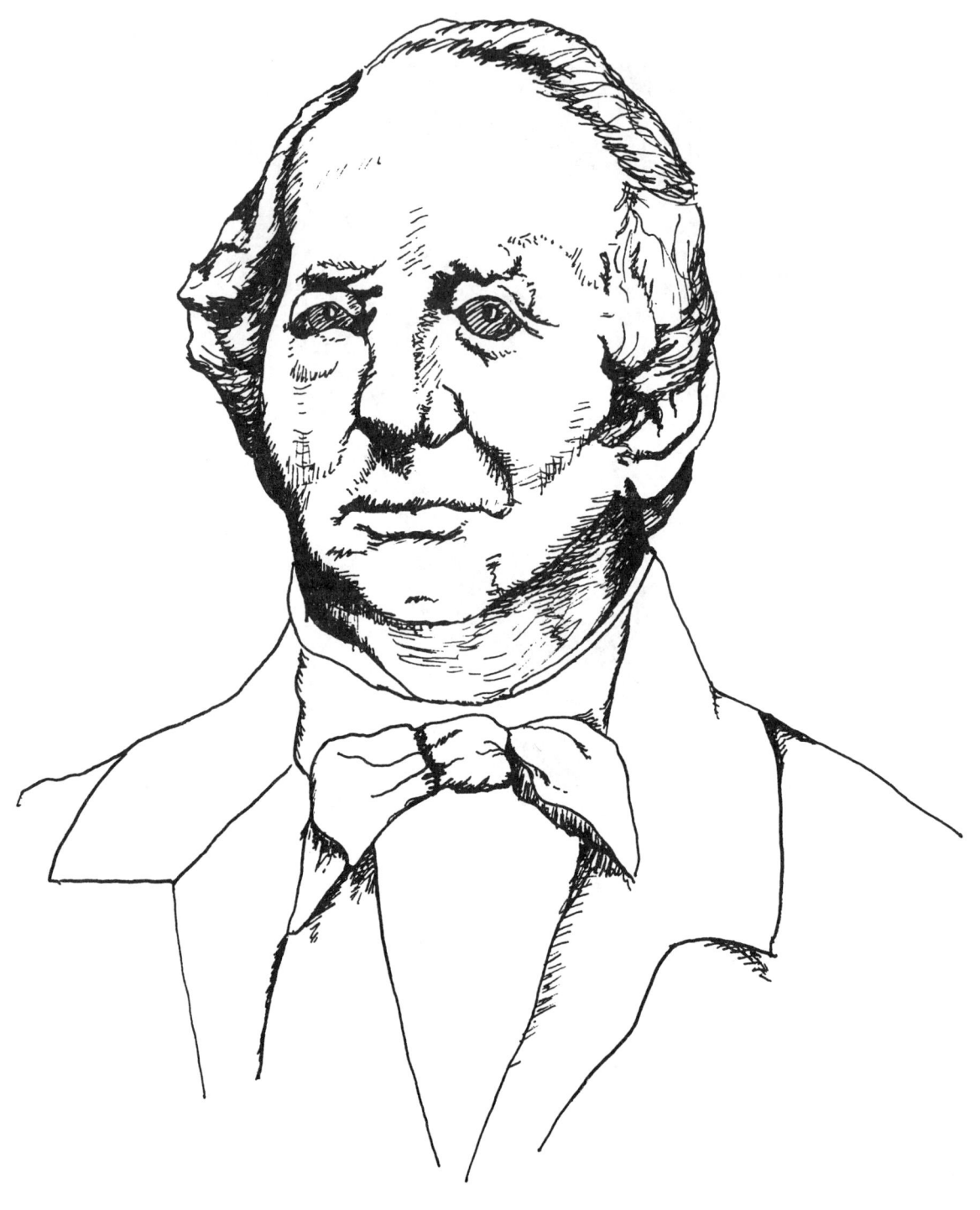

Bridges Beyond Sound
© 1996 Corinne K. Jensema
Paul H. Brookes Publishing Co., Inc.

S-19
Robert Davila

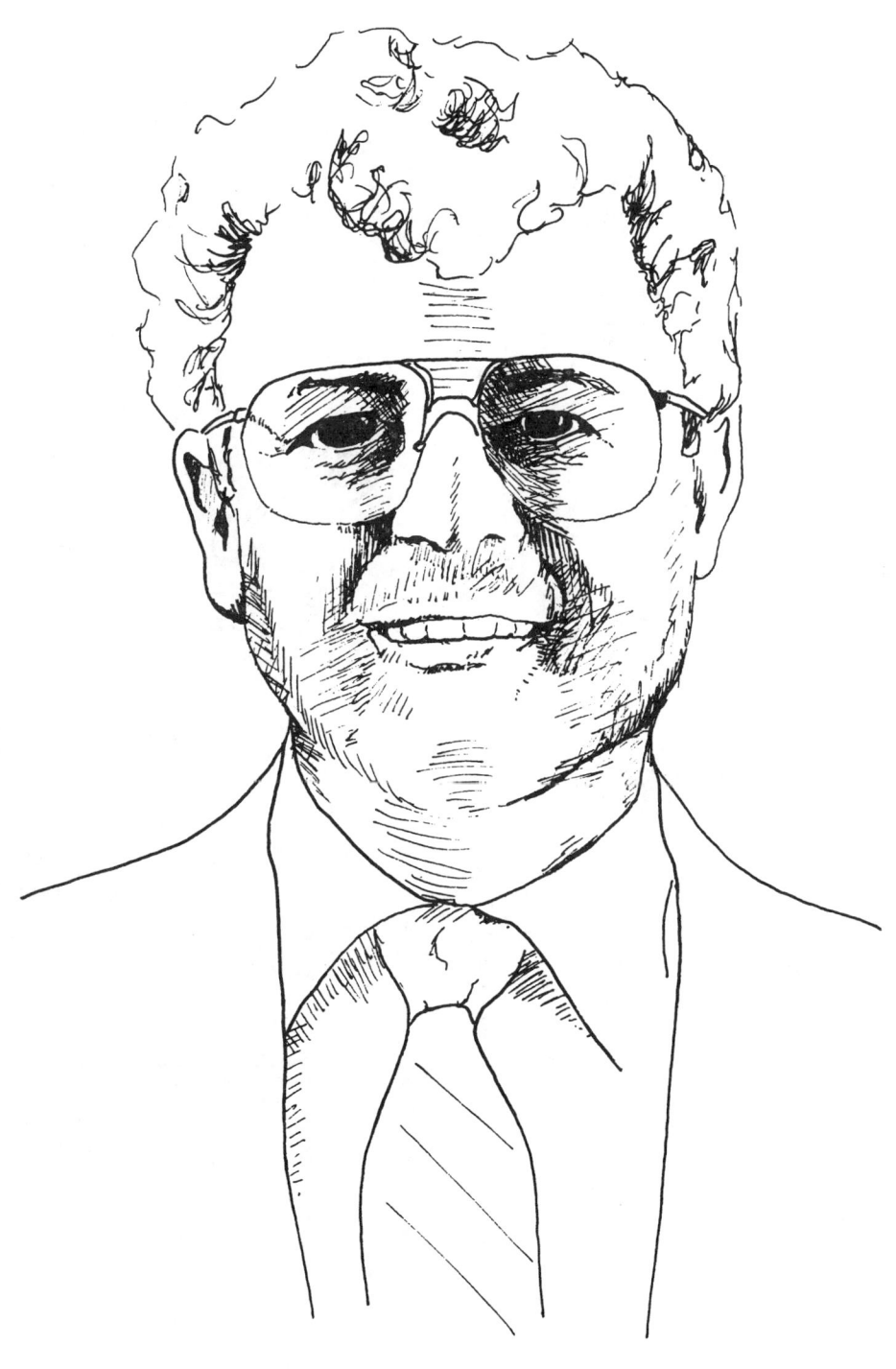

Bridges Beyond Sound
© 1996 Corinne K. Jensema
Paul H. Brookes Publishing Co., Inc.

S-19
LINDA BOVE

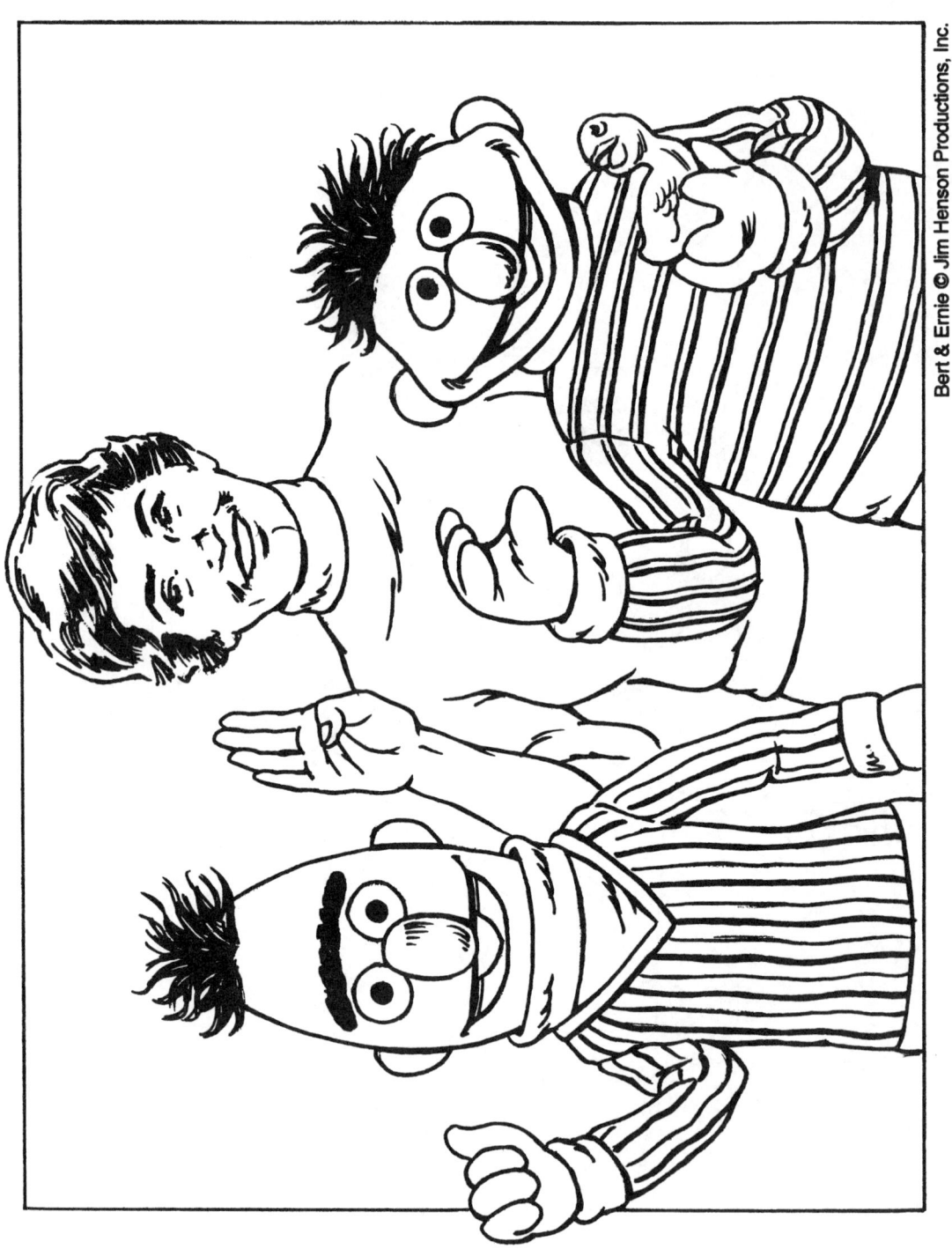

Bridges Beyond Sound
© 1996 Corinne K. Jensema
Paul H. Brookes Publishing Co., Inc.

S-19
MARLEE MATLIN

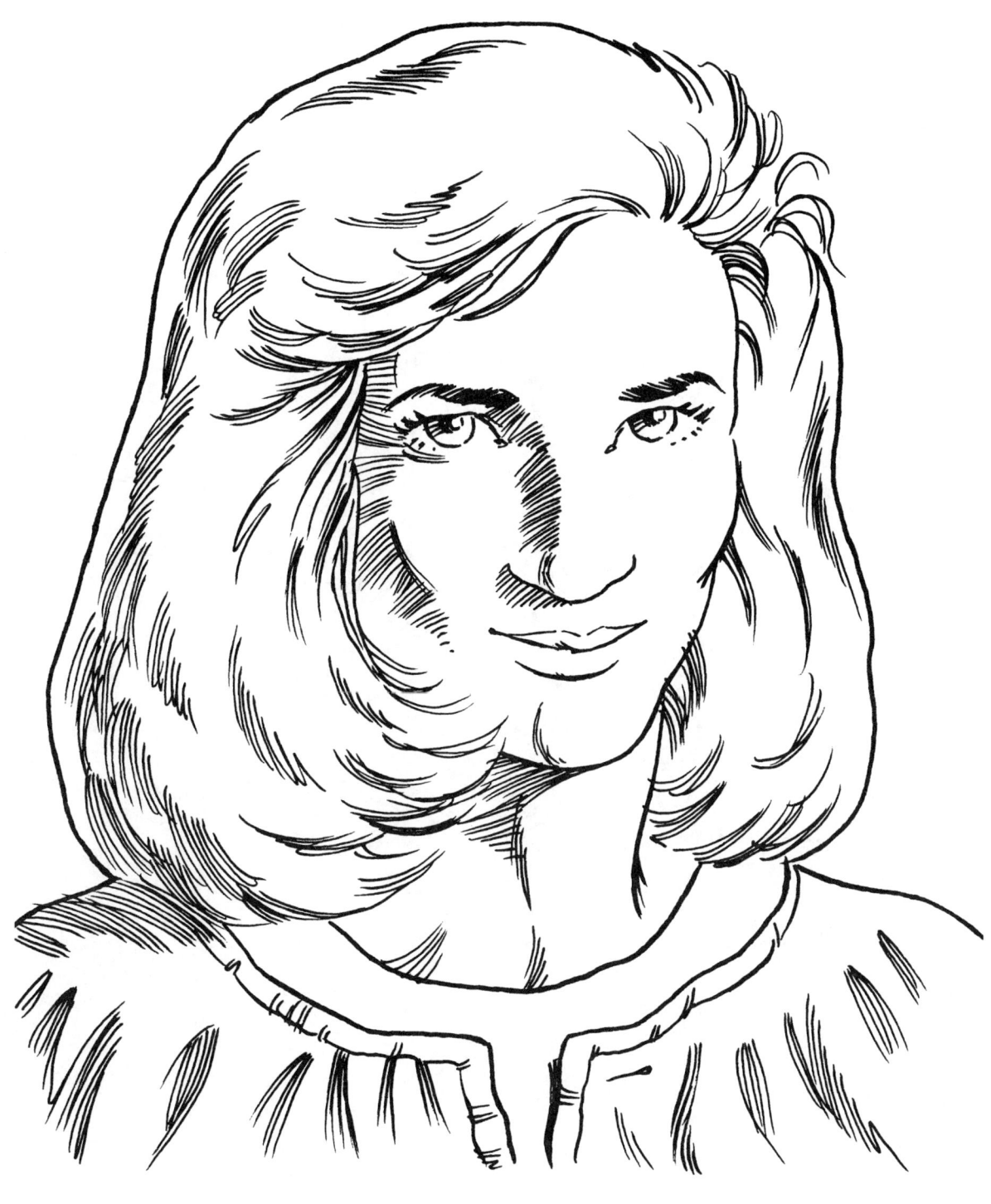

Bridges Beyond Sound
© 1996 Corinne K. Jensema
Paul H. Brookes Publishing Co., Inc.

S-19
Louis Frisino

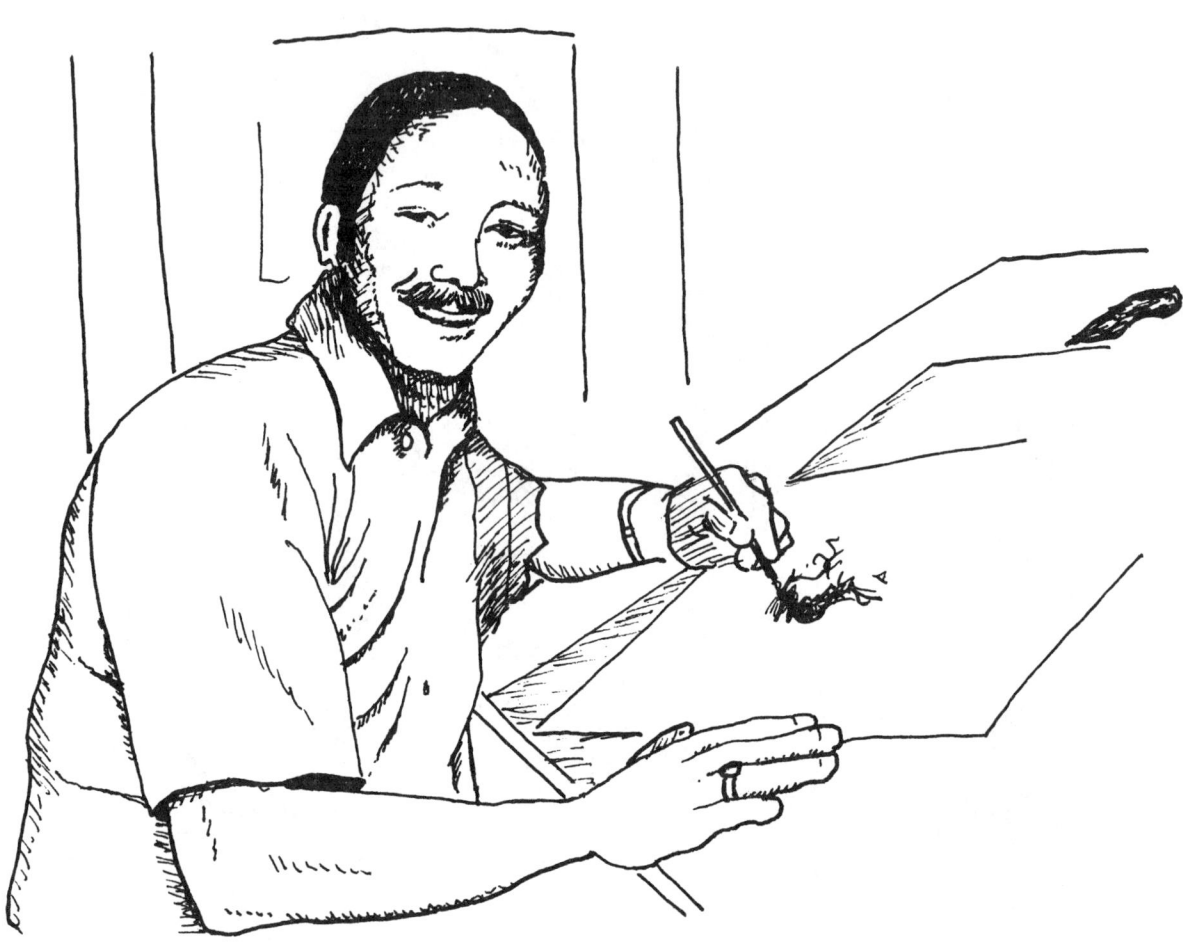

Bridges Beyond Sound
© 1996 Corinne K. Jensema
Paul H. Brookes Publishing Co., Inc.

S-19
I. [Irving] King Jordan

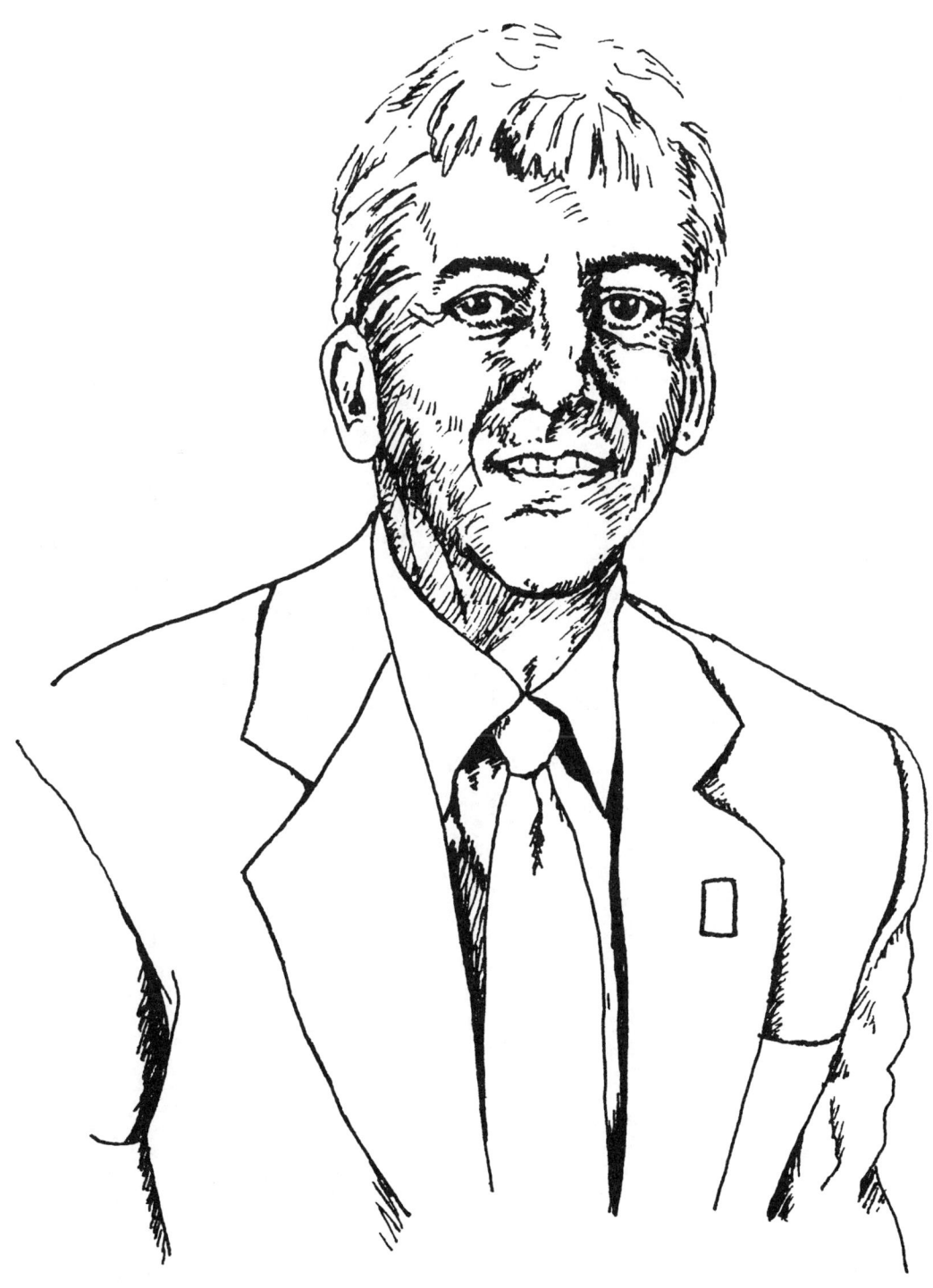

Bridges Beyond Sound
© 1996 Corinne K. Jensema
Paul H. Brookes Publishing Co., Inc.

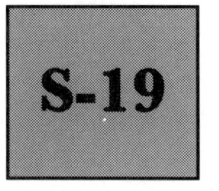

NELLIE WILLHITE

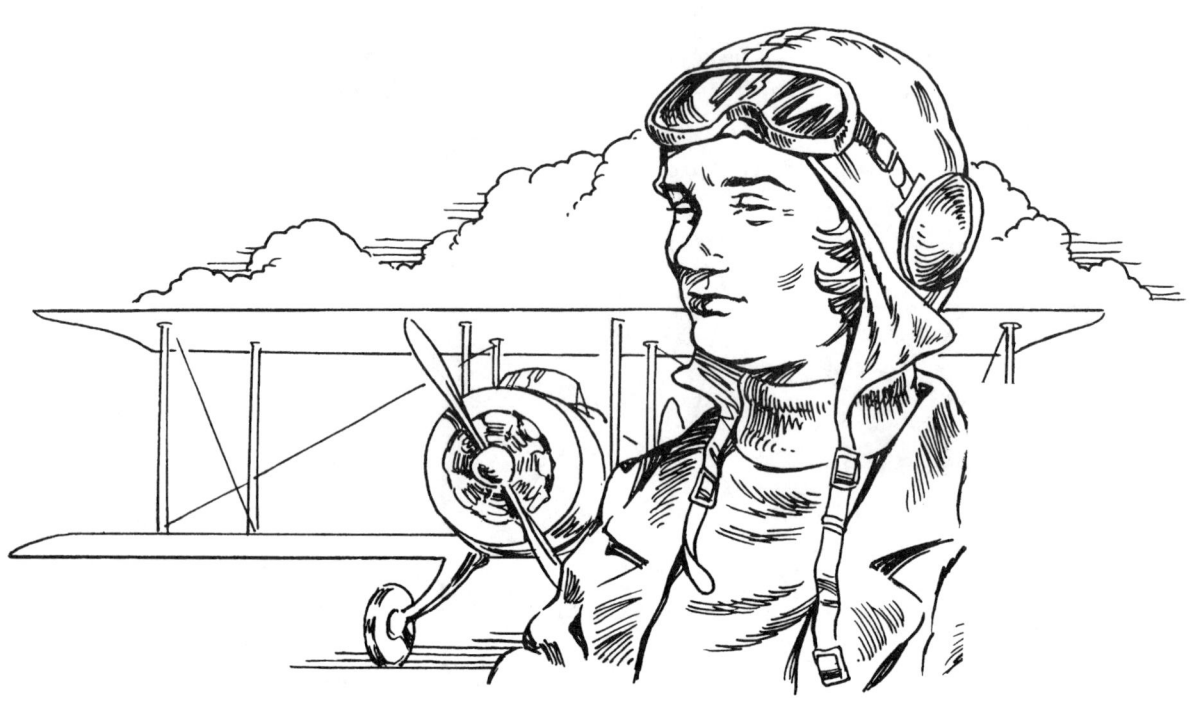

Bridges Beyond Sound
© 1996 Corinne K. Jensema
Paul H. Brookes Publishing Co., Inc.

S-19

Douglas Tilden

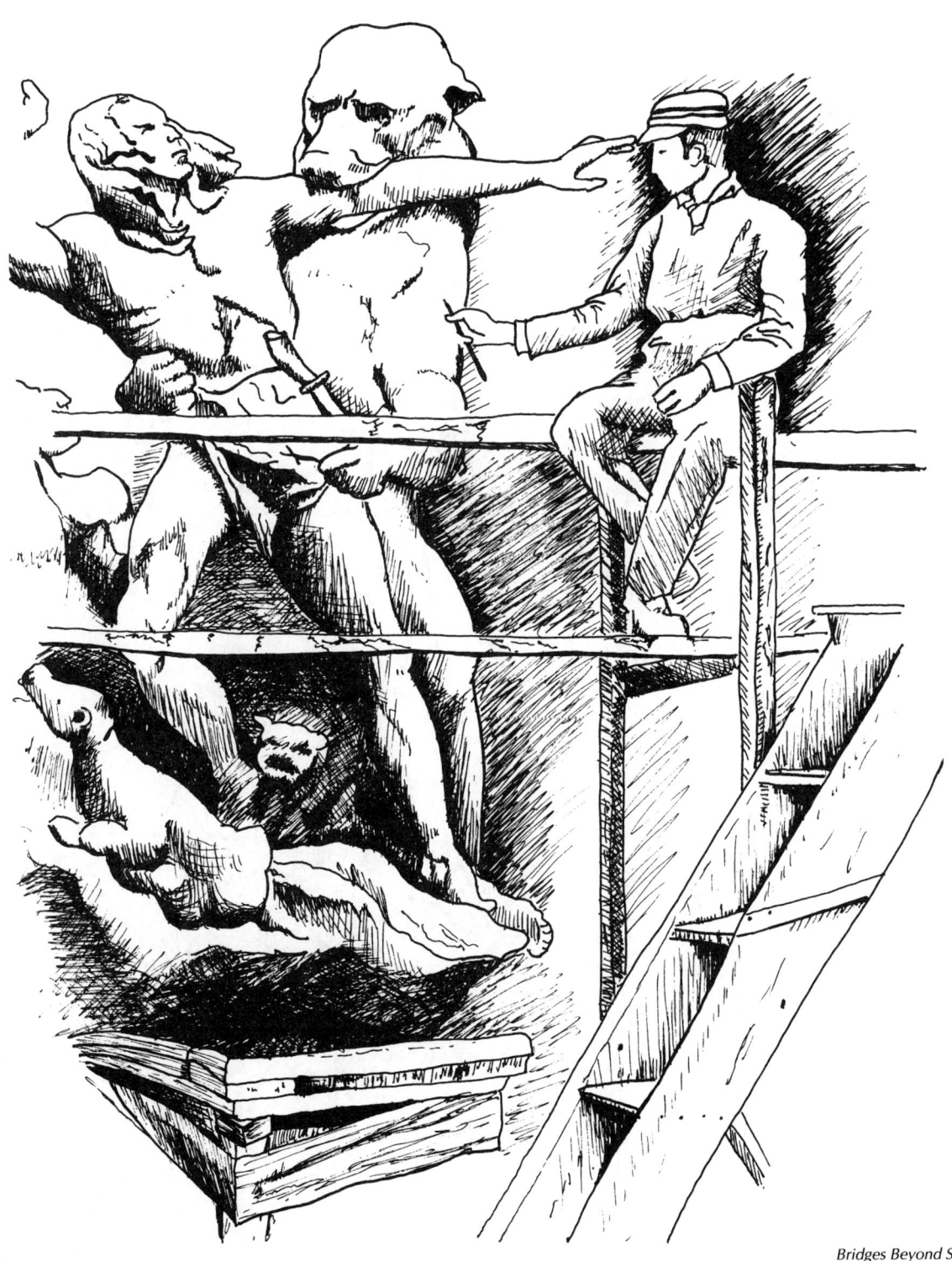

Bridges Beyond Sound
© 1996 Corinne K. Jensema
Paul H. Brookes Publishing Co., Inc.

S-19
JOHN CLARKE

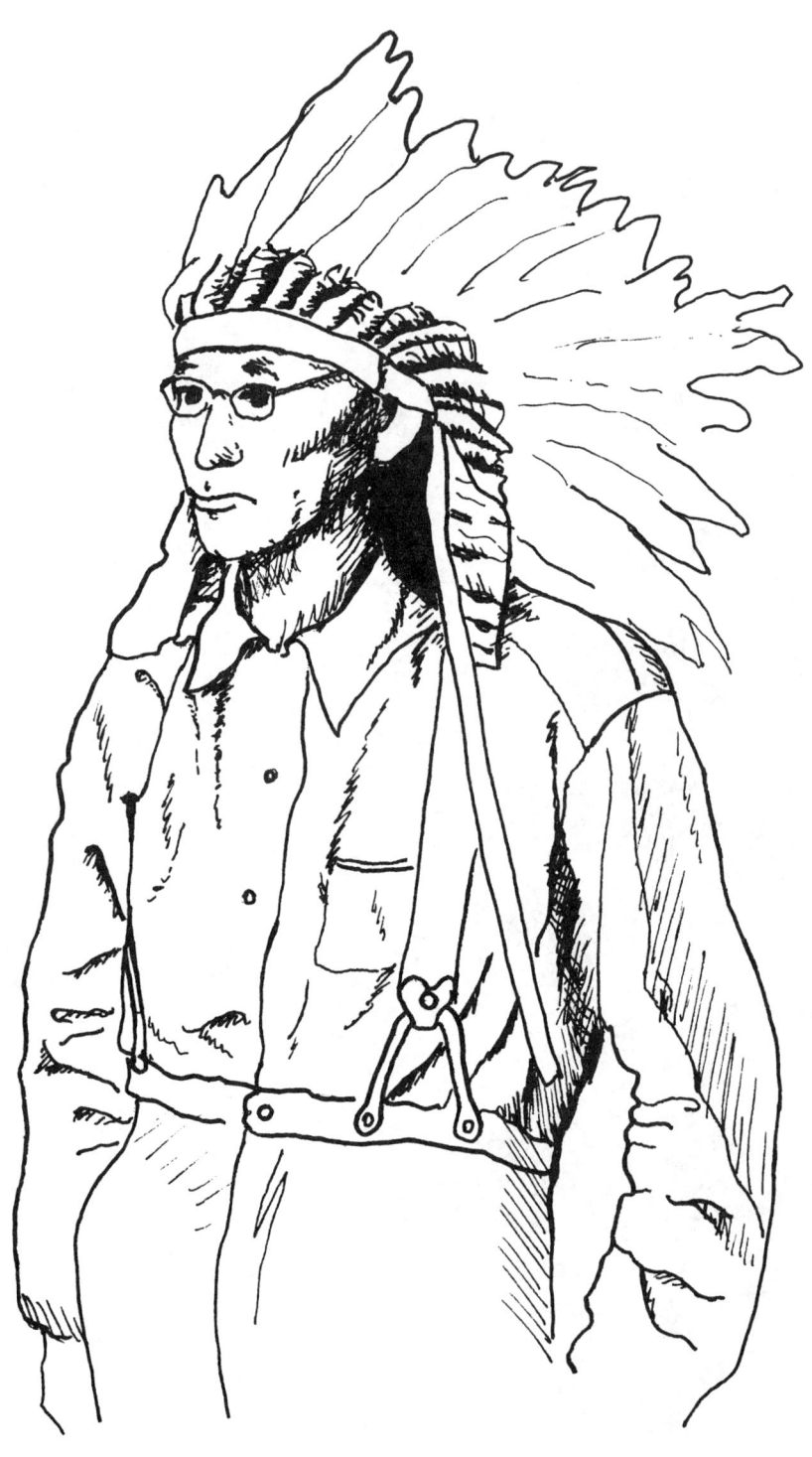

Bridges Beyond Sound
© 1996 Corinne K. Jensema
Paul H. Brookes Publishing Co., Inc.

S-19

HEATHER WHITESTONE

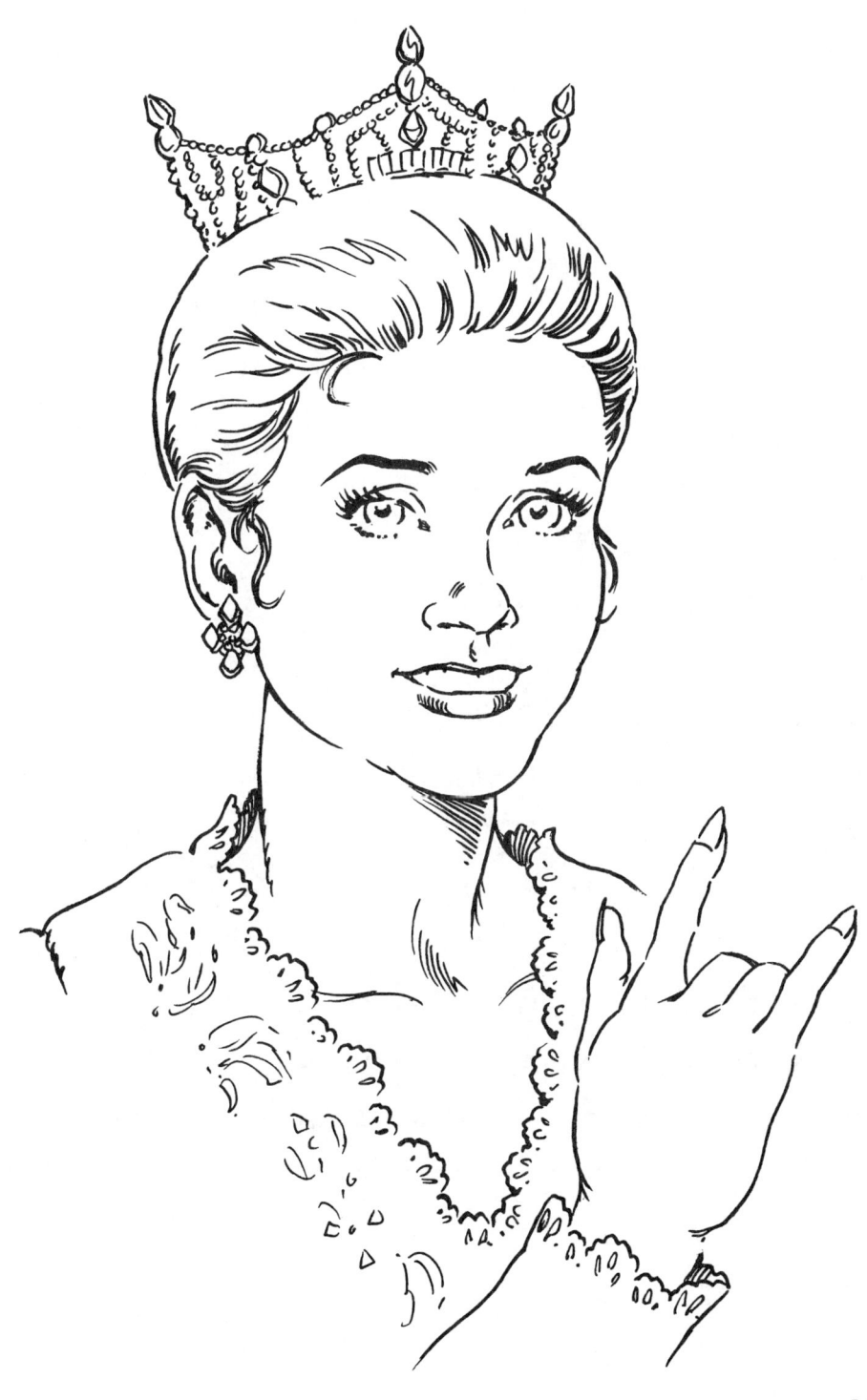

Bridges Beyond Sound
© 1996 Corinne K. Jensema
Paul H. Brookes Publishing Co., Inc.

S-20

WORD SEARCH: SUCCESSFUL PEOPLE WITH HEARING IMPAIRMENTS

Using the clues on the next page, identify each person. The 12 names are hidden in the puzzle. Words may appear horizontally, vertically, forward, or backward.

```
M L X E S M A O N I S I R F S I U O L A
A E I Z E N E N E D L I T S A L G U O D
R C K E R L R N N O X W J W Q N M Y U T
L R N E L L I E W I L L H I T E E T F P
E S O N L O C H C I M R E F I N N N E J
E L I K I T T Y O N E I L L S P A T R K
M K A T H Y B U C K L E Y E N I K S R O
A N C J J E C W R P L M N J I Y B G I R
T H O C U R T I S P R I D E B V B N G M
L C X Z A S L I N D A B O V E D F G N H
I E N O T S E T I H W R E H T A E H O Y
N I K I N G J O R D A N T R E W Q D L L
L A U R E N T C L E R C L O S R E B M E
F J O H N C L A R K E O T N A L A L E N
C J A R O X O N A L I V A D T R E B O R
D E A F S M I T H L E A H A R O K A R Y
```

Bridges Beyond Sound
© 1996 Corinne K. Jensema
Paul H. Brookes Publishing Co., Inc.

S-20

CLUES FOR WORD SEARCH

The answers to each of the clues below can be found in the word search. Words may appear horizontally, vertically, forward, or backward.

1. Pilot

2. Native American woodcarver

3. Californian sculptor

4. Soldier

5. *Sesame Street* member

6. President of Gallaudet University

7. America's first deaf teacher of the deaf

8. Actress

9. Former U.S. Assistant Secretary for Education

10. Comedienne

11. Maryland wildlife artist

12. Former Miss America

Bridges Beyond Sound
© 1996 Corinne K. Jensema
Paul H. Brookes Publishing Co., Inc.

S-20
ANSWER KEY

WORD SEARCH: SUCCESSFUL PEOPLE WITH HEARING IMPAIRMENTS

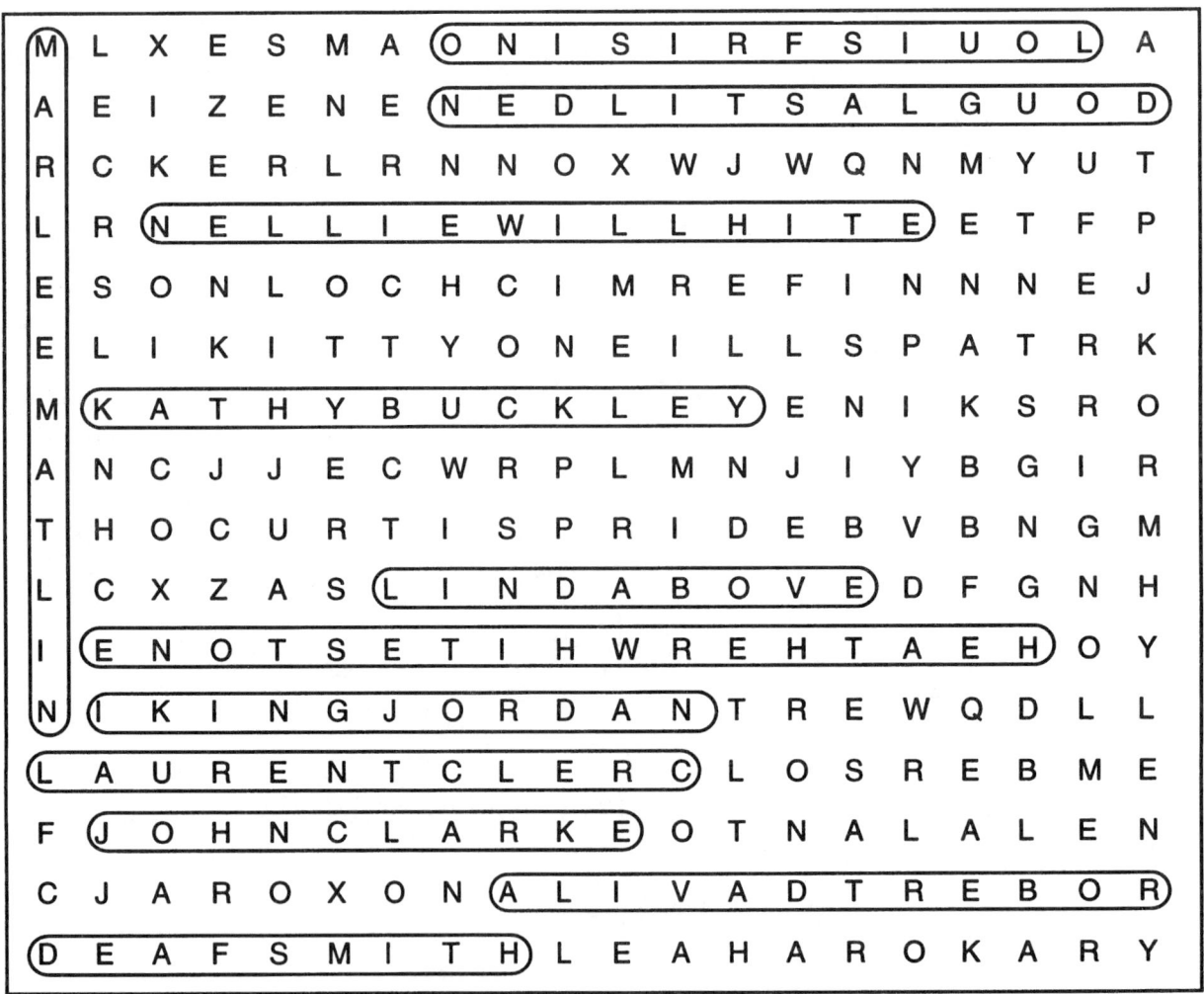

Bridges Beyond Sound
© 1996 Corinne K. Jensema
Paul H. Brookes Publishing Co., Inc.

S-20 ANSWER KEY

CLUES FOR WORD SEARCH

1. Pilot—***Nellie Willhite***
2. Native American woodcarver—***John Clarke***
3. Californian sculptor—***Douglas Tilden***
4. Soldier—***Deaf Smith***
5. *Sesame Street* member—***Linda Bove***
6. President of Gallaudet University—***I. King Jordan***
7. America's first deaf teacher of the deaf—***Laurent Clerc***
8. Actress—***Marlee Matlin***
9. Former U.S. Assistant Secretary for Education—***Robert Davila***
10. Comedienne—***Kathy Buckley***
11. Maryland wildlife artist—***Louis Frisino***
12. Former Miss America—***Heather Whitestone***

S-21
CHILDREN WITH AND WITHOUT HEARING IMPAIRMENTS PLAYING TOGETHER

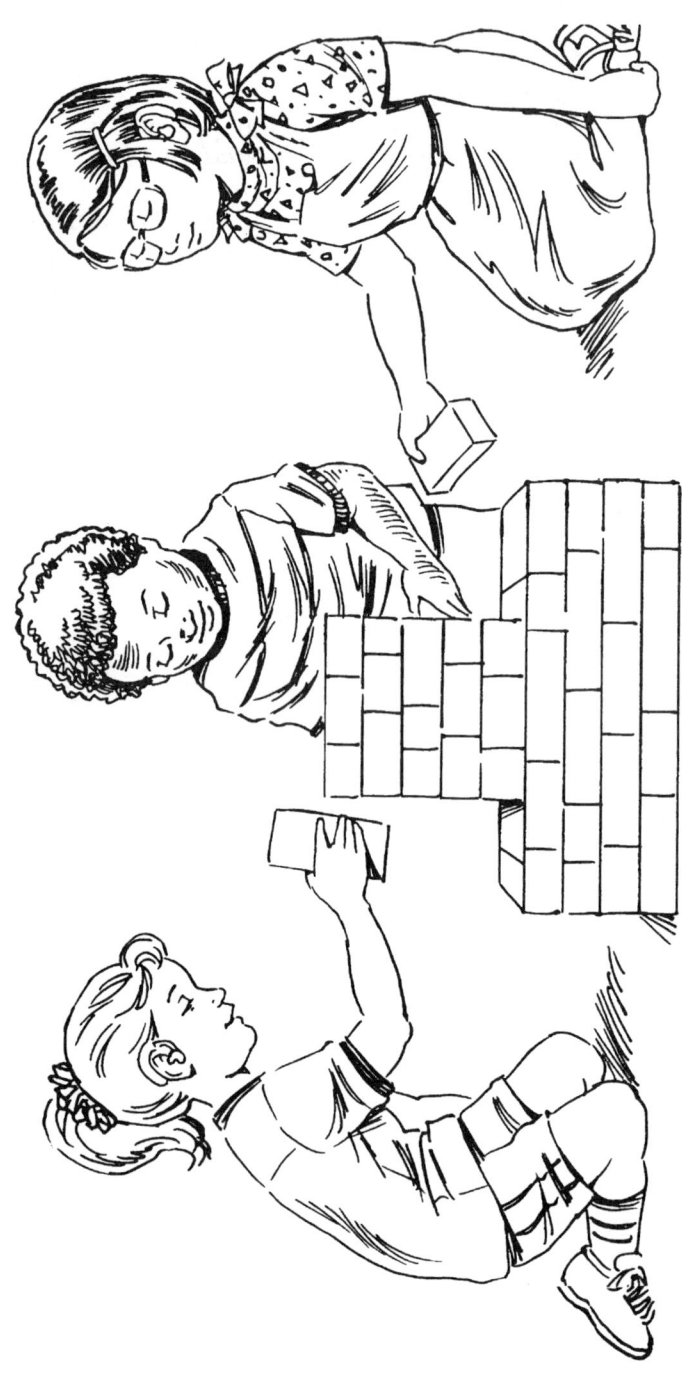

Bridges Beyond Sound
© 1996 Corinne K. Jensema
Paul H. Brookes Publishing Co., Inc.

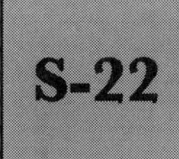

CROSSWORD PUZZLE

Below is a crossword puzzle using words that you have learned. Clues for the answers are found on the next page.

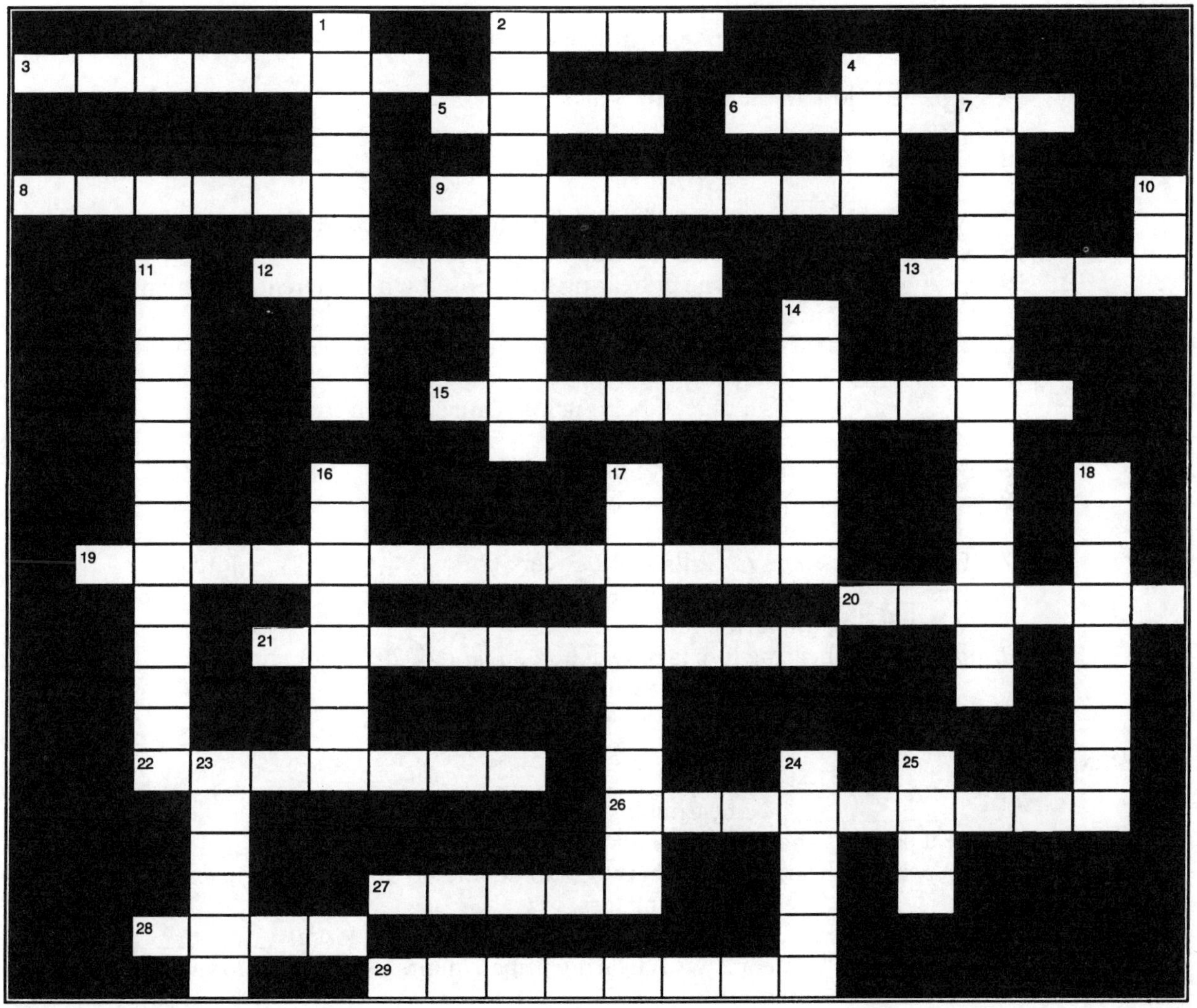

Bridges Beyond Sound
© 1996 Corinne K. Jensema
Paul H. Brookes Publishing Co., Inc.

S-22

CLUES FOR CROSSWORD PUZZLE

ACROSS

2. A person who has a hearing loss so severe that he or she cannot understand speech is _____ .
3. Twenty-four _____ people in the United States have some kind of hearing loss.
5. When sounds are over 130 dB, they can cause _____ .
6. If a person's hearing loss is between 15 dB and 25 dB, he or she has a _____ hearing loss.
8. The _____ of a hearing loss refers to the characteristics of the loss and cause.
9. A hearing loss that can occur or develop at any time during a person's life is _____ .
12. Deaf culture's form of handing down stories, events, games, and so forth is called _____ .
13. A hearing loss that is both conductive and sensorineural is called _____ .
15. A hearing loss that occurs naturally as people age is called _____ .
19. _____ is a type of hearing loss caused when there is a problem in the inner ear or auditory nerve.
20. The deaf actress who starred on the television show *Reasonable Doubts* is _____ Matlin.
21. _____ is a type of hearing loss caused when there is a problem in the outer or middle ear.
22. Degenerative hearing losses can be slow and _____ , or quick.
26. Congenital hearing losses can be _____ from your parents or grandparents.
27. The deaf president of Gallaudet University is _____ Jordan.
28. The _____ method promotes teaching speechreading to people with hearing impairments.
29. If a person's hearing loss is between 40 dB and 60 dB, he or she has a _____ hearing loss.

DOWN

1. _____ is a hearing loss that is present at birth.
2. Deaf people's shared history and heritage is called _____ .
4. If a person's hearing loss is between 25 dB and 40 dB, he or she has a _____ hearing loss.
7. A term to describe a person with any type of hearing loss is _____ .
10. A machine that people with hearing impairments use to communicate over the telephone is called _____ .
11. _____ is a method of determining what a person is saying by watching how his or her lips move.
14. _____ is the measurement of sound levels.
16. If a person's hearing loss is over 95 dB, he or she has a _____ hearing loss.

Bridges Beyond Sound
© 1996 Corinne K. Jensema
Paul H. Brookes Publishing Co., Inc.

S-22

17. A type of hearing loss that changes from day to day is called _____.
18. The quietest sound a person can hear is the _____.
23. Former Assistant Secretary for the U.S. Office of Special Education and Rehabilitative Services is _____ Davila.
24. If a person has a hearing loss between 65 dB and 95 dB, he or she has a _____ hearing loss.
25. Some people with hearing impairments use _____ language to communicate.

Bridges Beyond Sound
© 1996 Corinne K. Jensema
Paul H. Brookes Publishing Co., Inc.

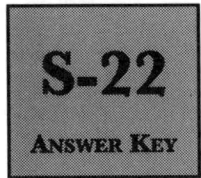

Crossword Puzzle

S-22
ANSWER KEY

CLUES FOR CROSSWORD PUZZLE

ACROSS

2. A person who has a hearing loss so severe that he or she cannot understand speech is **DEAF**.
3. Twenty-four **MILLION** people in the United States have some kind of hearing loss.
5. When sounds are over 130 dB, they can cause **PAIN**.
6. If a person's hearing loss is between 15 dB and 25 dB, he or she has a **SLIGHT** hearing loss.
8. The **NATURE** of a hearing loss refers to the characteristics of the loss and cause.
9. A hearing loss that can occur or develop at any time during a person's life is **ACQUIRED**.
12. Deaf culture's form of handing down stories, events, games, and so forth is called **SIGNLORE**.
13. A hearing loss that is both conductive and sensorineural is called **MIXED**.
15. A hearing loss that occurs naturally as people age is called **PRESBYCUSIS**.
19. **SENSORINEURAL** is a type of hearing loss caused when there is a problem in the inner ear or auditory nerve.
20. The deaf actress who starred on the television show *Reasonable Doubts* is **MARLEE** Matlin.
21. **CONDUCTIVE** is a type of hearing loss caused when there is a problem in the outer or middle ear.
22. Degenerative hearing losses can be slow and **GRADUAL**, or quick.
26. Congenital hearing losses can be **INHERITED** from your parents or grandparents.
27. The deaf president of Gallaudet University is **I. KING** Jordan.
28. The **ORAL** method promotes teaching speechreading to people with hearing impairments.
29. If a person's hearing loss is between 40 dB and 60 dB, he or she has a **MODERATE** hearing loss.

DOWN

1. **CONGENITAL** is a hearing loss that is present at birth.
2. Deaf people's shared history and heritage is called **DEAF CULTURE**.
4. If a person's hearing loss is between 25 dB and 40 dB, he or she has a **MILD** hearing loss.
7. A term to describe a person with any type of hearing loss is **HEARING IMPAIRED**.
10. A machine that people with hearing impairments use to communicate over the telephone is called **TDD**.
11. **SPEECHREADING** is a method of determining what a person is saying by watching how his or her lips move.
14. **DECIBEL** is the measurement of sound levels.
16. If a person's hearing loss is over 95 dB, he or she has a **PROFOUND** hearing loss.
17. A type of hearing loss that changes from day to day is called **FLUCTUATING**.
18. The quietest sound a person can hear is the **THRESHOLD**.
23. Former Assistant Secretary for the U.S. Office of Special Education and Rehabilitative Services is **ROBERT** Davila.

Bridges Beyond Sound
© 1996 Corinne K. Jensema
Paul H. Brookes Publishing Co., Inc.

S-22 ANSWER KEY

24. If a person has a hearing loss between 65 dB and 95 dB, he or she has a **SEVERE** hearing loss.
25. Some people with hearing impairments use **SIGN** language to communicate.

S-23

POSTTEST

This is a test to see how much you know now that you have learned about people who have hearing impairments. Follow the instructions for each part of this test.

Circle the letter next to the right answer.

1. People who are deaf _____ .

    a. are all old.

    b. can be any age.

    c. all became deaf before they were born.

    d. all became deaf from listening to rock music too loudly.

2. Children who are deaf _____ .

    a. all go to their neighborhood schools.

    b. all go to schools only for deaf students.

    c. only are in classes for deaf children in their neighborhood schools.

    d. can go to any school where they can get special services.

3. Children who are deaf _____ .

    a. can have parents who are deaf or who can hear.

    b. only have parents who are deaf.

    c. only have parents who can hear.

    d. do not have parents.

4. All children who are deaf _____ .

    a. can speechread well.

    b. know sign language.

    c. wear hearing aids.

    d. need special help to communicate with hearing people.

Bridges Beyond Sound
© 1996 Corinne K. Jensema
Paul H. Brookes Publishing Co., Inc.

S-23

5. _____ is a famous person who is deaf.

   a. Mr. Rogers

   b. Linda Bove

   c. Michael Jordan

   d. Michael Jackson

6. The machine that helps people who are deaf use the telephone is called a _____ .

   a. VCR.

   b. TV.

   c. TDD.

   d. Ph.D.

7. The part of a hearing aid that you put in your ear is called _____ .

   a. an antenna.

   b. a cord.

   c. a listener.

   d. an ear mold.

8. The sign language used in the United States is called _____ .

   a. American Sign Language.

   b. USA Sign Language.

   c. English Sign Language.

   d. Hand Sign Language.

9. The chart used when measuring hearing is called _____ .

   a. an audiogram.

   b. a sound level chart.

   c. a hearing status indicator.

   d. a hearing loss graph.

Bridges Beyond Sound
© 1996 Corinne K. Jensema
Paul H. Brookes Publishing Co., Inc.

S-23

10. The outer part of your ear is called the _____ .

   a. earring holder.
   b. eardrum.
   c. cochlea.
   d. pinna.

Decide whether each sentence is true or false. Circle the correct response.

1. People who are deaf can drive.   True   False
2. People who are deaf always have deaf children.   True   False
3. People who are deaf always marry other people who are deaf.   True   False
4. People who are deaf can become teachers.   True   False
5. People can lose their hearing from accidents.   True   False
6. Hearing aids can help all people who are deaf.   True   False
7. A former Miss America is deaf.   True   False
8. It is easy to speechread.   True   False
9. The sign language we use in the United States came from France.   True   False
10. The first deaf teacher of the deaf in the United States was Deaf Smith.   True   False

Write your answers after each question.

1. If a student in your class was deaf and the interpreter did not show up for class one day, how could you help that student communicate in class?

Bridges Beyond Sound
© 1996 Corinne K. Jensema
Paul H. Brookes Publishing Co., Inc.

S-23

2. If your class is having a party and everyone is to bring something, how could you tell a classmate who is deaf what to bring and what everyone else is bringing?

Bridges Beyond Sound
© 1996 Corinne K. Jensema
Paul H. Brookes Publishing Co., Inc.

INDEX

Acquired hearing loss, 25, 28, 35, 36, 84, 86
ADA, *see* Americans with Disabilities Act of 1990
Age at onset of hearing loss, 28, 36, 86
Air-conduction testing, 26, 36, 90
Alarm clocks, 96
Alerting devices, 10, 34, 36, 97
Alexander Graham Bell Association for the Deaf, Inc., 56
American Academy of Otolaryngology–Head and Neck Surgery, 56
American Athletic Association of the Deaf, 56
American Deafness and Rehabilitation Association, 56–57
American Hearing Research Foundation, 57
American Manual Alphabet, 109
American Sign Language (ASL), 12–13, 31, 36, 47, 88–89, 107–108
American Society for Deaf Children, 57
American Speech-Language-Hearing Association (ASHA), 57
Americans with Disabilities Act (ADA) of 1990, PL 101-336, 47, 117
Amplifier, 36
Answering door, 34, 97
Anvil, 36, 93
Appearance of people with hearing impairments, 4–5
ASHA, *see* American Speech-Language-Hearing Association
ASL, *see* American Sign Language
Assistive technology references, 51
Association of Late-Deafened Adults, 58
Attitudes toward deaf people, 12
Audiogram, 26, 36, 84, 90–92
Audiological testing, 25–26, 84
 air-conduction testing, 26, 36, 90
 bone-conduction testing, 26, 37, 90
Audiologist, 84
Auditory nerve, 93
Aural (oral) method, 30–31, 40, 87–88, 115

Baby cry detector, 97
Bell, Alexander Graham, 116
Better Hearing Institute, 58
Bicycling, 34
Biographies on deaf people, 49, 119–123
Bone-conduction testing, 26, 37, 90
Bove, Linda, 12, 120–121, 128

Buckley, Kathy, 119, 124

Captioned Films for the Deaf, 117
Causes of hearing loss, 5, 25, 28, 35
Childbearing, 35
Children of deaf adults (CODAs), 13
Clarke, John, 115, 122–123, 134
Clarke School for the Deaf, 115
Clerc, Laurent, 114, 120, 126
Closed captioning, 11, 37, 97–98, 117–118
Cochlea, 37, 93
CODAs, *see* Children of deaf adults
Communication
 alerting devices, 10, 34, 36, 97
 alternate methods of, 6, 13–17, 20–21, 33
 cued speech, 32, 37, 89
 education for, 30–32
  manual method, 31–32, 40, 88–89
  oral method, 30–31, 40, 87–88, 115
 within family, 10–11, 32, 88
 interpreters, 19, 39–40, 47–48, 106
 language development, 6–7, 27–28, 30, 85
 problem solving for, 15–17
 in school, 19
 sign language, 12–13, 31–32, 88–89
 simultaneous communication, 32, 89
 speech, 6–7, 30–31, 33, 87–88
 speechreading, 6, 8–9, 30, 42
 telephone use, 11, 34, 42–46, 96–97, 117
 television viewing, 11, 37, 40, 97–98, 117–118
 tips for, 106
 total communication, 32, 42, 89
Communication assistants, 97
Conductive hearing loss, 26, 37, 84
Conference of Educational Administrators Serving the Deaf, 58
Congenital hearing loss, 25, 28, 35, 37, 83, 86
Connect-the-dots exercises, 99–102
Convention of American Instructors of the Deaf, 58
Crossword puzzles, 141–146
Cued speech, 32, 37, 89

Dancing, 33
Davila, Robert, 120, 127
dB, *see* Decibel
Deaf Artists of America, Inc., 58–59

Deaf community, 29, 35, 87
Deaf culture, 5, 11–13, 25, 29, 31, 35, 37–38, 83, 87
   reference materials on, 50–51
Deaf education, 30–32, 87
   reference materials on, 49–50
Deaf humor, 29, 87
Deafness, 6
   definition of, 25, 37, 83
   negative connotation of, 25, 83
   see also Hearing loss
Deafness and Communicative Disorders Branch, 59
Deafness Research Foundation, 59
Deafpride, Inc., 59
Decibel (dB), 38, 84
Decoders, 38, 98, 117–118
Degenerative hearing loss, 28, 38, 86
Degree of hearing loss, 27, 84–85
Diagnosis of hearing loss
   audiological testing, 25–26, 84
   early, 30
   screening for, 8
Down syndrome, 5
Driving, 33

Ear canal, 38, 93
Ear structure and function, 93–95
Earache, 93
Eardrum, 38, 93
Earmold, 38
Education for All Handicapped Children Act of 1975, PL 94-142, 117
Education of children with hearing impairments, 19, 30–32, 35, 87
   history of, 114–118
   manual method, 31–32, 40, 88–89
   oral (aural) method, 30–31, 40, 87–88, 115
   see also Schools
Effects of hearing loss, 27–28, 85–86
Emotional effects of hearing loss, 29, 86
Engelsman, Bernard, 115
Episcopal Conference of the Deaf, 60
Eustachian tube, 38, 93

Facts about deafness, 4, 77–80
Families, 10–11
   with all deaf members, 11
   communication within, 32, 88
   containing a deaf member, 10–11
Fingerspelling, 38, 108–111
Fluctuating hearing loss, 28, 39, 86
Fraternal Society of the Deaf, 116
Frisino, Louis, 121, 130

Gallaudet, Thomas Hopkins, 114
Gallaudet University, 115, 118, 121
Games, 35, 140
Getting the attention of a deaf person, 10, 34
Glossary, 36–42
Gregg, John R., 116

Hammer, 39, 93
Hard-of-hearing, 5, 83
Hearing aids, 7–8, 96
   behind-the-ear, 96
   body aids, 96
   definition of, 39, 96
   in-the-ear, 96
Hearing Information Center, 60
Hearing loss
   acquired, 25, 28, 35, 36, 84, 86
   age at onset of, 28, 36, 86
   attitudes toward people with, 12
   causes of, 35
   congenital, 25, 28, 35, 37, 83, 86
   definition of, 25
   degrees of, 27, 84–85
   diagnosis of, 25–26, 84
   education of children with, 30–32
   effects of, 27–28, 85–86
   emotional effects of, 29, 86
   evaluating instructional materials for depictions of people with, 68
   facts and myths about, 4, 77–80
   hereditary, 5, 10, 35, 39
   high- versus low-frequency, 6, 9
   identifying people with, 4–5
   incidence of, 3, 25, 83
   nature of, 28, 85–86
   noise-induced, 5
   among older people, 25, 28
   other disabilities and, 29, 86
   types of, 26–27, 84
   see also Deafness
Hearing Loss Link, 60–61
Hearing screening, 8
Hearing threshold, 26, 27, 39, 84
Hereditary deafness, 5, 10, 35, 39
Heritage of deaf people, 11–12; *see also* Deaf culture
Hertz (Hz), 39, 84
High-frequency hearing loss, 6, 9
History of the deaf in the United States, 114–118
Hubbard, Gardiner G., 115
Humming, 6
Humor, 29, 87
Hz, *see* Hertz

IDEA, *see* Individuals with Disabilities Education Act of 1990, PL 101-476
Identifying people with hearing loss, 4–5
Incidence of hearing loss, 3, 25, 83
Inclusion, 39, 66–67
Individuals with Disabilities Education Act (IDEA) of 1990, PL 101-476, 25
Inner ear, 93
Institute for Disabilities Research and Training, Inc., 61
Interactive videotape transcript, 3–22
International Catholic Deaf Association, 61
International Lutheran Deaf Association, 61
Interpreters, 19, 39–40, 47–48
   notetaking by, 47

oral, 47
   sign, 47
   tips for use of, 47–48, 106

Jordon, I. King, 12, 118, 121–122, 131

Knapp, Frederick, 115

Language development, 6–7, 27–28, 30, 85; see also Speech
Light signals, 10, 34, 96, 97
Lipreading, see Speechreading
Low-frequency hearing loss, 6

Manual method, 31–32, 40, 88–89
Manually Coded English (MCE), 47
Matlin, Marlee, 32, 121, 129
MCE, see Manually Coded English
Middle ear, 93
Mild hearing loss, 27, 40, 85, 91
Mixed hearing loss, 27, 40, 84
Moderate hearing loss, 27, 40, 85, 91
Morse, Samuel, 115
Music
   hearing loss induced by loudness of, 5
   listening to by people with hearing impairments, 33
Myths about deafness, 4, 77–80

National Association of the Deaf, 61, 116
National Black Deaf Advocates, 62
National Congress of Jewish Deaf, 62
National Cued Speech Association, 62
National Fraternal Society of the Deaf, 62
National Information Center on Deafness, 62–63
National Institute on Deafness and Other Communication Disorders Information Clearinghouse, 63
National organizations for the deaf, 56–65
National Technical Institute for the Deaf, 63, 117
National Theater of the Deaf, 117
Noises
   audiogram of environmental and speech sounds, 92
   hearing loss induced by, 5
   made by hearing aids, 7–8
   made by people with hearing impairments, 34
Normal hearing, 27, 40, 85, 91
Notetaking, 47

Older people, 25, 28, 41, 84, 86
Open captioning, 40
Oral (aural) method, 30–31, 40, 87–88, 115
Organizations for the deaf
   history of, 116
   national and international, 56–65
   state, 52–55
Outer ear, 93

Permanent hearing loss, 28, 40, 86
Pidgin Signed English (PSE), 40, 47, 107–108
Pinna, 41, 93
PL 94-142, see Education for all Handicapped Children Act of 1975
PL 101-336, see Americans with Disabilities Act (ADA) of 1990
PL 101-431, see Television Decoder Circuitry Act of 1990
PL 101-476, see Individuals with Disabilities Education Act (IDEA) of 1990
Play, 35, 140
Posttest, 147–149
Presbycusis, 28, 41, 86
Pretest, 71–76
Profound hearing loss, 27, 41, 85, 91
PSE, see Pidgin Signed English

Reference materials, 49–51
   for children, 112–113
Registry of Interpreters for the Deaf, Inc., 47, 63, 117
Residual hearing, 41
Round window, 93

Schools, 19, 35
   inclusion in, 39, 66–67
   interpreters in, 47
   tips for evaluating instructional materials, 68
   worksheets for use in, see Worksheets for students
   see also Education of children with hearing impairments
SEE, see Signed Exact English
Self Help for Hard of Hearing People, Inc., 64
Sensorineural hearing loss, 26–27, 41, 84
Sesame Street, 12, 13, 110, 120–121, 128
Severe hearing loss, 27, 41, 85, 91
Sign language, 12–13, 31–32, 88–89, 107–108
   reference materials on, 50
   see also specific types of signing
Signed Exact English (SEE), 41
Signlore, 29, 41, 87
Simultaneous communication, 32, 89
Slight hearing loss, 27, 41, 85, 91
Smith, Erastus "Deaf," 119–120, 125
Sound perception, 93
Speech
   audiogram of speech sounds, 92
   cued, 32, 37, 89
   explaining how speech sounds are made, 6
   of people with hearing impairments, 6–7, 33
   teaching to people with hearing impairments, 30–31, 87–88
Speechreading, 6, 8–9, 30, 42, 106
Sports, 56, 117
State organizations for the deaf, 52–55, 116
Stirrup, 42, 93

Successful people with hearing impairments, 119–139

TDD, *see* Telecommunication device for the deaf
Telecommunication device for the deaf (TDD), 11, 34, 42–46, 96–97, 117
    abbreviations used with, 44–45
    handling interruptions with, 46
    making calls with, 43
    receiving calls with, 43
    state relay service for, 97
    transmission problems with, 43–44
Telecommunications for the Deaf, Inc., 64
Telegraph, 115
Telephone, 11, 34, 42–46, 96–97, 117
Teletypewriter (TTY), 42, 117
Television, 11
    closed-captioned, 11, 37, 97–98, 117–118
    open-captioned, 40
Television Decoder Circuitry Act, PL 101-431, 117
Temporary hearing loss, 28, 42, 86
Terminology, 36–42
Text telephone (TT), 42
The Ear Foundation, 60
Tilden, Douglas, 122, 133
Total communication, 32, 42, 89
TT, *see* Text Telephone
TTY, *see* Teletypewriter
Tubes placed in ear, 93

Tympanic membrane, 38, 93
Types of hearing loss, 26–27, 84
    conductive, 26, 37, 84
    mixed, 27, 40, 84
    sensorineural, 26–27, 41, 84

Vibrations, 6, 93
Videotape transcript, 3–22
Volta Bureau, 116

Whitestone, Heather, 123, 135
Willhite, Nellie, 122, 132
Word jumble, 103–105
Word pronunciation, 6–7
Word search, 136–139
Worksheets for students
    connect-the-dots, 99–102
    crossword puzzles, 141–146
    ear structure, 94–95
    facts and myths about deafness, 77–80
    fingerspelling, 110–111
    posttest, 147–149
    pretest, 71–76
    word jumble, 103–105
    word search, 136–139
    world without sound, 81–82
World Federation of the Deaf, 64
World Recreation Association of the Deaf, Inc., 65